W9-BPJ-667

READER'S DIGEST

GUIDE TO

MEDICAL CURES & TREATMENTS

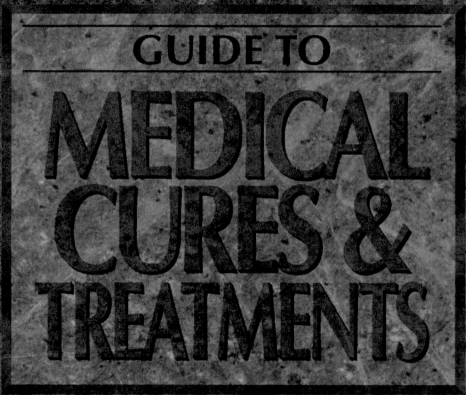

The Reader's Digest Association (Canada) Ltd.
Montreal

STAFF

Project Editors
Gayla Visalli
Andrew R. Byers

Art Associates
Barbara Lapic
John McGuffie
Cécile Germain

Research Editor
Wadad Bashour

Copy Preparation
Gilles Humbert

Coordinator
Susan Wong

Production
Holger Lorenzen

CONTRIBUTORS

Editorial Director
Genell J. Subak-Sharpe

Art Editor
Judy Speicher

Writers and Editors
Diana Benzaia
Susan Carleton
Catherine Caruthers
Mark Deitch
Diane Goetz
Ann Forer
Jennifer Freeman
Helene MacLean
Emily Paulsen
Sharon Pestka
Sarah Subak-Sharpe
Luba Vikhanski

Technical Assistant
Christel Henning

Medical Editors
Morton D. Bogdonoff, M.D.
Valerie Ulene, M.D.

Medical Consultants
Raul Artal, M.D.
Nancy Barone, D.C.
Philip M. Kasofsky, M.D.
Mathew H.M. Lee, M.D.
George D. Roston, D.D.S.

Illustrators
Enid Hatton — Medical
Ray Skibinski — Herbal

Researchers/Technical Support

Arlyn Apollo
Mikola De Roo
JoAnn Ford
Gabby Immerman
Carl Li
Briar Lee Mitchell
Reem Nasser
Letta Neely
Debra Rabinowitz
Dushan G. Lukic

Photo Research
PhotoSearch, Inc.

Text Inputting
Niche Electronic Publishing

Index
Judy Yelon

Canadian Cataloguing in Publication Data

Main entry under title:

Reader's Digest guide to medical cures & treatments: a complete A-to-Z sourcebook of medical treatments, alternative opinions, and home remedies

Includes index.
ISBN 0-88850-518-3

1. Therapeutics—Popular works. I. Reader's Digest Association (Canada). II. Title: Guide to medical cures & treatments.

RC81.R43 1996   616   C95-900866-7

The acknowledgments and credits that appear on page 480 are hereby made a part of this copyright page.

Printed in Canada
96 97 98 99 / 5 4 3 2 1

TABLE OF CONTENTS

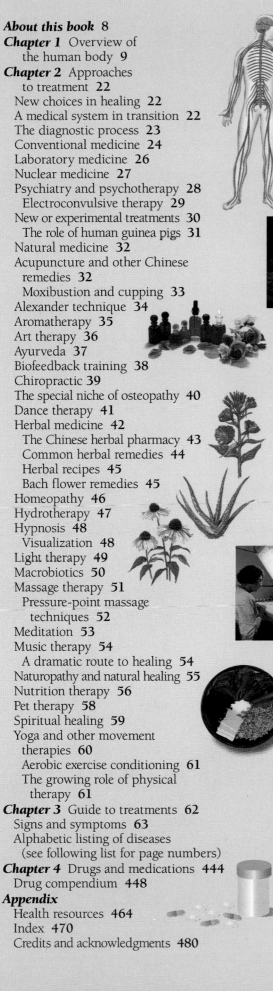

Directory of Diseases Covered in This Book

Many diseases have several names; some are used mostly by doctors, while others are part of everyday language. For example, myocardial infarction, heart attack, and coronary thrombosis all refer to the same disorder. The alphabetical directory below lists the most common terms for the diseases covered in this book. The index starting on page 490 has an even more complete listing.

TABLE OF CONTENTS

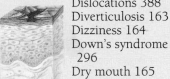
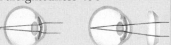
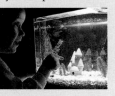
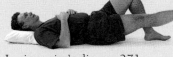

TABLE OF CONTENTS

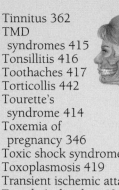

ABOUT THIS BOOK

In today's world, wise people are prepared to make informed decisions regarding their own and their family's health. This means knowing not only about diseases and how they are treated, but also what effect nutritional and lifestyle habits have in preventing illness. Is a particular medical problem something you can handle yourself? If not, how do you decide whom to consult? By using this handy A-to-Z medical reference, you will quickly find the information you need.

But the GUIDE TO MEDICAL CURES & TREATMENTS offers you much more than the usual home medical reference. It begins with an illustrated section on the human body that presents an overview of the various organ systems and how they work together. This is followed by a comprehensive survey of today's health-care system, which describes what to expect from various medical disciplines and provides insight into diagnostic and medical decision-making processes, as well as the domains of various medical specialties and the role of new and experimental treatments. A section on natural medicine covers dozens of alternative therapies—from acupuncture to yoga. You'll learn how these practices evolved, how to distinguish between reputable practitioners and charlatans, and what the advantages and shortcomings are of different alternative approaches.

The heart of the book—the A-to-Z section—is densely filled with information on the symptoms and diagnostic methods of more than 450 common diseases and disorders, how they are treated by both conventional and alternative medical practitioners, and what steps you can take to care for yourself. You'll also find lists of questions that you might want to ask your doctor, plus case histories (included with a number of entries), which are based on real patients; only their names have been changed to protect their privacy.

Following the A-to-Z section is a compendium of the most commonly used prescription and over-the-counter medications. Easy-to-use tables list generic and brand names for each drug, tell what it's used for, and give the major side effects and any precautions you should take while on the medication. Lastly, there is a directory of health resources that lists addresses and phone numbers of nearly 300 organizations, associations, and self-help or support groups.

This book was created by a team of medical educators and practitioners working with skilled medical writers and illustrators to ensure that the text is accurate, up-to-date, and understandable. Throughout, full-color illustrations and photographs are used to make the text even more meaningful.

We believe that no other home medical reference offers so much information on such a range of health problems and their treatments. And no other text allows you to compare conventional treatments, alternative therapies, and self-treatment in such an objective, straightforward presentation. The GUIDE TO MEDICAL CURES & TREATMENTS may well become the most important book in your home health library.

—The Editors

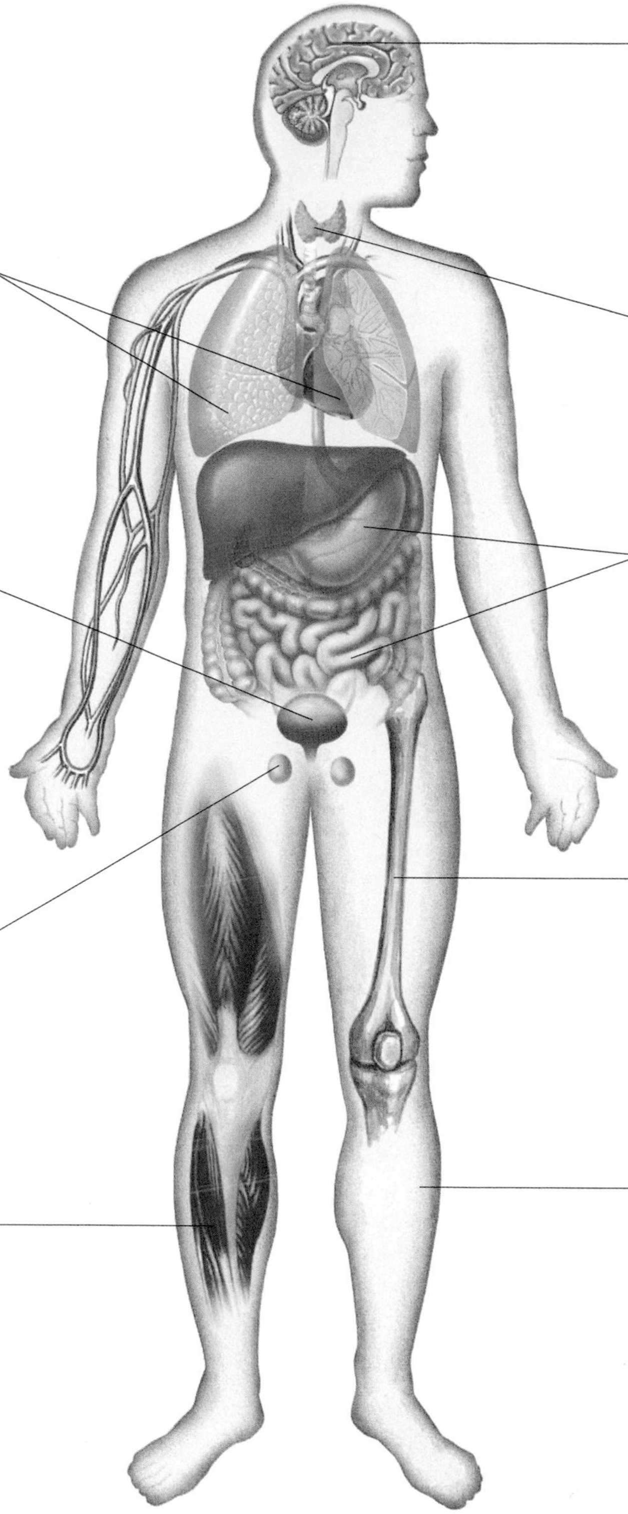

The brain, spinal cord, and peripheral nerves that make up the nervous system function as the body's communications network. The nervous system controls all other organ systems; it also is linked directly with the eyes, ears, and other sensory organs.

The respiratory and circulatory systems work in concert to provide a constant supply of oxygen to every cell in the body.

The endocrine system is made up of various glands that secrete hormones, the chemical messengers that control every bodily process. Hormones are also produced by such other organs as the stomach, lungs, kidneys, and heart.

The renal system filters wastes from the blood, which are then excreted through the urinary tract. The kidneys also produce hormones that are instrumental in controlling blood pressure and the manufacturing of red blood cells.

The organs of the digestive system form a hollow tube that extends form the mouth to the anus. As food passes through this tube, the various organs break it down into molecules that the body can turn into energy and new tissue.

The reproductive organs do more than ensure the survival of the species by producing future generations; they also make the hormones that give males and females their respective physical characteristics.

The adult skeleton contains more than 200 bones, giving the body its form and ability to move. Bones also store calcium and other essential minerals and serve as manufacturing plants for blood cells.

The body's 600 or 800 voluntary muscles work with the skeletal and nervous systems to make movement possible. Involuntary muscles are instrumental in the smooth functioning of all the other body systems.

The skin acts as a protective barrier against a hostile outside environment. It also manufactures vitamin D, helps regulate body temperature, and is essential to the sense of touch.

Philosophers and scientists alike have observed that human beings and other forms of animal life are made up of the same elements found in ordinary soil and water. But when these 20 or so basic elements combine in thousands of different ways to form a human body, the result is one of the most complex organisms on the planet and a never-ending source of both wonderment and mystery.

About 75 to 80 percent of an adult's body consists of slightly salty water; the rest is made up of chemical compounds, many of them unique to human beings. These various compounds are arranged to form hundreds of different kinds of cells, the body's smallest, most basic units.

All human life begins with the fusing of two cells, and the subsequent division and multiplication of cells to form a complete body follows the same general blueprint even though no two people are exactly alike. The average body contains 80 to 100 trillion cells, each programmed to grow, carry out a specific function, and even replicate itself. But, with the exception of blood cells, none function independently; instead, similar cells join together to form specific types of tissue—muscle, nerve, bone, and so forth. Each body organ is made up of a collection of related tissues. Finally, organs are organized into the different body systems illustrated above and on the following pages.

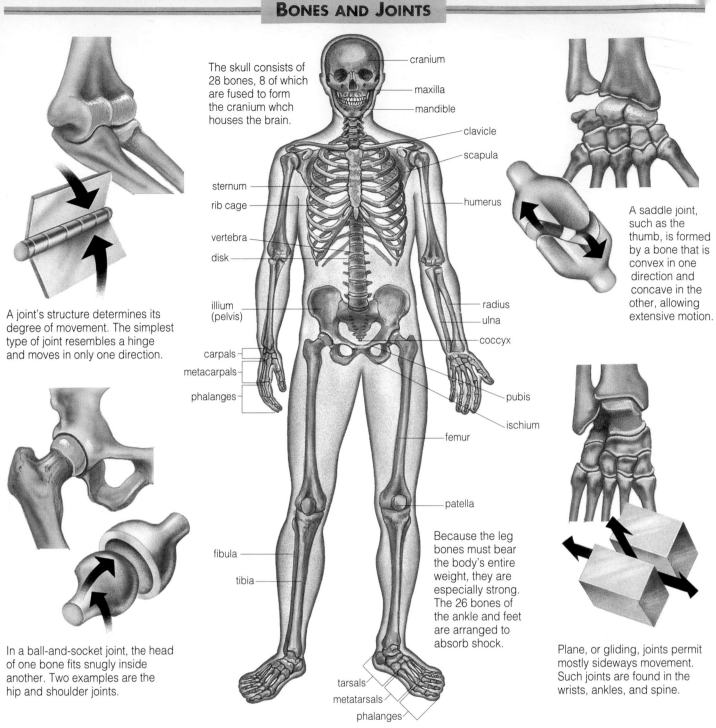

The skull consists of 28 bones, 8 of which are fused to form the cranium whch houses the brain.

cranium

maxilla

mandible

clavicle

scapula

sternum

rib cage

vertebra

disk

humerus

illium (pelvis)

radius

ulna

coccyx

carpals

metacarpals

phalanges

pubis

ischium

femur

patella

fibula

tibia

tarsals

metatarsals

phalanges

A joint's structure determines its degree of movement. The simplest type of joint resembles a hinge and moves in only one direction.

In a ball-and-socket joint, the head of one bone fits snugly inside another. Two examples are the hip and shoulder joints.

A saddle joint, such as the thumb, is formed by a bone that is convex in one direction and concave in the other, allowing extensive motion.

Because the leg bones must bear the body's entire weight, they are especially strong. The 26 bones of the ankle and feet are arranged to absorb shock.

Plane, or gliding, joints permit mostly sideways movement. Such joints are found in the wrists, ankles, and spine.

The human skeleton is an engineering marvel with numerous functions: Not only does it give the body its needed support and a protective framework for vital internal organs, but it also serves as a storehouse for calcium and other essential minerals and is critical in making new blood cells. Although we tend to regard bones as being inert, in reality they are in a constant state of flux and also change dramatically over a lifetime. At birth, a baby has about 350 bones, a number of which are soft and pliable. As the child grows, the bones harden and many, such as those in the skull, fuse together.

The typical adult skeleton has 206 bones and weighs only about 20 pounds. Ounce for ounce, however, compact bone tissue is one of nature's strongest materials. A cubic inch of bone can bear 19,000 pounds, making it four times stronger than reinforced concrete. Bones derive their incredible strength from their honeycombed structure and composition of calcium, phosphorus, and other mineral salts held together by collagen fibers. Nerves and blood vessels permeate the honeycombed structure and calcium and other minerals constantly move in and out of bone tissue. New blood cells are continually being made in the marrow, the spongy interior.

Cartilage, a tough, slippery material, covers the ends of bones, cushioning the joints and reducing friction. Ligaments act as bindings to keep bones in place, and tendons attach muscles to the bones. To permit movement, bones act as levers, the joints are fulcrums, and muscles contract to provide the necessary force (see facing page).

Age takes its toll on bones and joints. The knees and hips are especially vulnerable to degenerative arthritis. And with advancing age, bones begin to lose some of their calcium, making them porous and weak, a condition called osteoporosis (page 320).

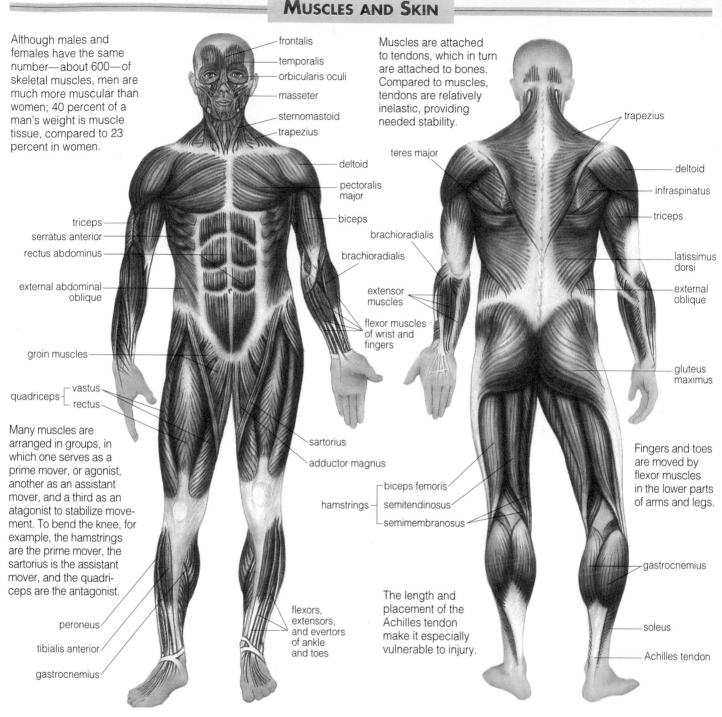

Although males and females have the same number—about 600—of skeletal muscles, men are much more muscular than women; 40 percent of a man's weight is muscle tissue, compared to 23 percent in women.

frontalis
temporalis
orbicularis oculi
masseter
sternomastoid
trapezius

deltoid
pectoralis major
biceps

triceps
serratus anterior
rectus abdominus

external abdominal oblique

groin muscles

quadriceps — vastus
— rectus

Many muscles are arranged in groups, in which one serves as a prime mover, or agonist, another as an assistant mover, and a third as an atagonist to stabilize movement. To bend the knee, for example, the hamstrings are the prime mover, the sartorius is the assistant mover, and the quadriceps are the antagonist.

peroneus
tibialis anterior
gastrocnemius

sartorius
adductor magnus

flexors, extensors, and evertors of ankle and toes

Muscles are attached to tendons, which in turn are attached to bones. Compared to muscles, tendons are relatively inelastic, providing needed stability.

teres major

brachioradialis

brachioradialis

extensor muscles

flexor muscles of wrist and fingers

trapezius

deltoid
infraspinatus
triceps

latissimus dorsi

external oblique

gluteus maximus

Fingers and toes are moved by flexor muscles in the lower parts of arms and legs.

biceps femoris
hamstrings — semitendinosus
semimembranosus

The length and placement of the Achilles tendon make it especially vulnerable to injury.

gastrocnemius

soleus

Achilles tendon

The body contains three types of muscle: cardiac, found only in the heart; involuntary smooth muscles, which are part of various organs; and the skeletal muscles, which are attached to bones and make voluntary movement possible.

Skeletal muscles—the body's most abundant tissue—are made up of bundles of long fibers bound together by connective tissue. Each fiber is surrounded by tiny capillaries, which deliver a steady supply of oxygen needed for the muscles to function. The fibers in a particular muscle remain constant in number throughout life, but they enlarge when exercised frequently and shrink, or atrophy, with disuse and age.

Every set of muscles is served by one or more nerves. Movement occurs when nerve signals set off specific chemical reactions that cause certain muscles to contract. Most muscle disorders are actually due to nerve problems. The muscle weakness of multiple sclerosis is one example.

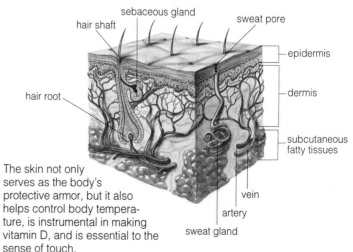

sebaceous gland
hair shaft
sweat pore

epidermis

hair root

dermis

subcutaneous fatty tissues

vein

artery

sweat gland

The skin not only serves as the body's protective armor, but it also helps control body temperature, is instrumental in making vitamin D, and is essential to the sense of touch.

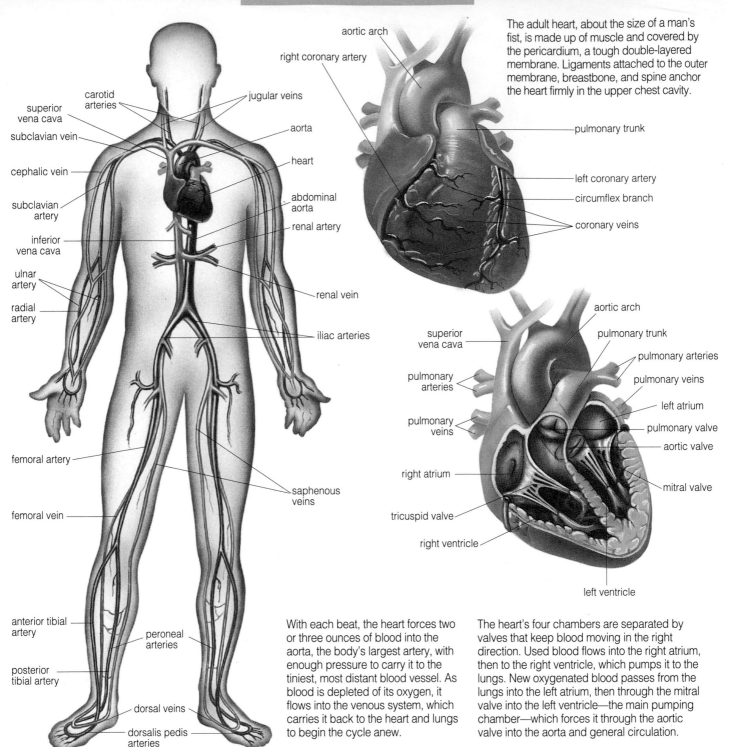

aortic arch

right coronary artery

carotid arteries

superior vena cava

subclavian vein

cephalic vein

subclavian artery

inferior vena cava

ulnar artery

radial artery

femoral artery

femoral vein

anterior tibial artery

peroneal arteries

posterior tibial artery

dorsal veins

dorsalis pedis arteries

jugular veins

aorta

heart

abdominal aorta

renal artery

renal vein

iliac arteries

saphenous veins

The adult heart, about the size of a man's fist, is made up of muscle and covered by the pericardium, a tough double-layered membrane. Ligaments attached to the outer membrane, breastbone, and spine anchor the heart firmly in the upper chest cavity.

pulmonary trunk

left coronary artery

circumflex branch

coronary veins

aortic arch

superior vena cava

pulmonary trunk

pulmonary arteries

pulmonary veins

pulmonary arteries

pulmonary veins

left atrium

pulmonary valve

aortic valve

right atrium

mitral valve

tricuspid valve

right ventricle

left ventricle

With each beat, the heart forces two or three ounces of blood into the aorta, the body's largest artery, with enough pressure to carry it to the tiniest, most distant blood vessel. As blood is depleted of its oxygen, it flows into the venous system, which carries it back to the heart and lungs to begin the cycle anew.

The heart's four chambers are separated by valves that keep blood moving in the right direction. Used blood flows into the right atrium, then to the right ventricle, which pumps it to the lungs. New oxygenated blood passes from the lungs into the left atrium, then through the mitral valve into the left ventricle—the main pumping chamber—which forces it through the aortic valve into the aorta and general circulation.

The adult body has some 60,000 miles of blood vessels that supply oxygen and other nutrients to every cell and carry away carbon dioxide and other wastes. The heart, one of nature's most durable pumps, constantly circulates 8 to 10 pints of blood through this vast network. On a typical day, the heart beats more than 100,000 times, pumping out 2,600 gallons of blood. This adds up to more than 2.5 billion heartbeats over an average lifetime, with never more than a fraction of a second's rest between each beat.

Although the heart is designed to last a lifetime, cardiovascular disease remains our leading cause of death, claiming about a million lives a year in North America. Most of these deaths are due to heart attacks, often in the prime of life. It is estimated that more than 60 million North Americans suffer from a cardiovascular disorder, with high blood pressure and coronary artery disease the most prevalent. These disorders are epidemic world wide, concentrated mostly in developed nations. They are a relatively modern phenomenon that experts attribute to a combination of lifestyle factors (for example, eating a high-fat diet, smoking, not exercising) and heredity. Increasingly, however, researchers are showing that heart attacks, strokes, and other cardiovascular events can be prevented by adopting a prudent, heart-healthy lifestyle (see Angina, page 79, and Heart Attack, page 216).

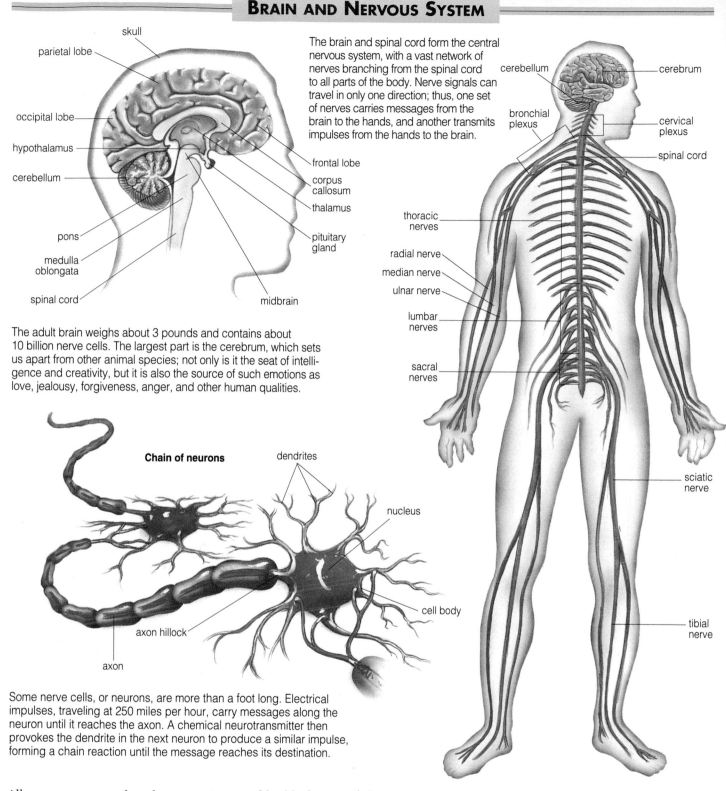

The brain and spinal cord form the central nervous system, with a vast network of nerves branching from the spinal cord to all parts of the body. Nerve signals can travel in only one direction; thus, one set of nerves carries messages from the brain to the hands, and another transmits impulses from the hands to the brain.

Brain diagram labels: skull, parietal lobe, occipital lobe, hypothalamus, cerebellum, pons, medulla oblongata, spinal cord, midbrain, pituitary gland, thalamus, corpus callosum, frontal lobe

Body diagram labels: cerebellum, cerebrum, bronchial plexus, cervical plexus, spinal cord, thoracic nerves, radial nerve, median nerve, ulnar nerve, lumbar nerves, sacral nerves, sciatic nerve, tibial nerve

The adult brain weighs about 3 pounds and contains about 10 billion nerve cells. The largest part is the cerebrum, which sets us apart from other animal species; not only is it the seat of intelligence and creativity, but it is also the source of such emotions as love, jealousy, forgiveness, anger, and other human qualities.

Chain of neurons — dendrites, nucleus, cell body, axon hillock, axon

Some nerve cells, or neurons, are more than a foot long. Electrical impulses, traveling at 250 miles per hour, carry messages along the neuron until it reaches the axon. A chemical neurotransmitter then provokes the dendrite in the next neuron to produce a similar impulse, forming a chain reaction until the message reaches its destination.

All our movements, thoughts, sensations, and bodily functions are controlled by the brain and nervous system, the most highly evolved among all living creatures and the least understood. Neuroscientists are only beginning to unravel the myriad mysteries of the human brain, and many predict we will never fully understand so many of the things we take for granted: memory, language, creativity, and so forth.

Taken as a whole, the nervous system is actually a complex branching network of systems with many overlapping parts and functions, all controlled by the brain and its spinal cord extension. Such automatic, or involuntary, functions as breathing, circulation, and digestion are directed largely by

the autonomic nervous system, which is divided into the sympathetic and parasympathetic components. In simplified terms, these two systems act as switches to turn organs on and off, thus maintaining a state of balance.

Superficial sensory nerves receive messages from the outside world and transmit them to the brain, where they are interpreted and sent back through the body via the cranial or spinal nerves. All this takes only a split second and often requires little or no thought. However, when something goes awry with the brain or other componenets of the nervous system, manifestations can be disastrous, ranging from trivial movement disorders to paralysis and dementia.

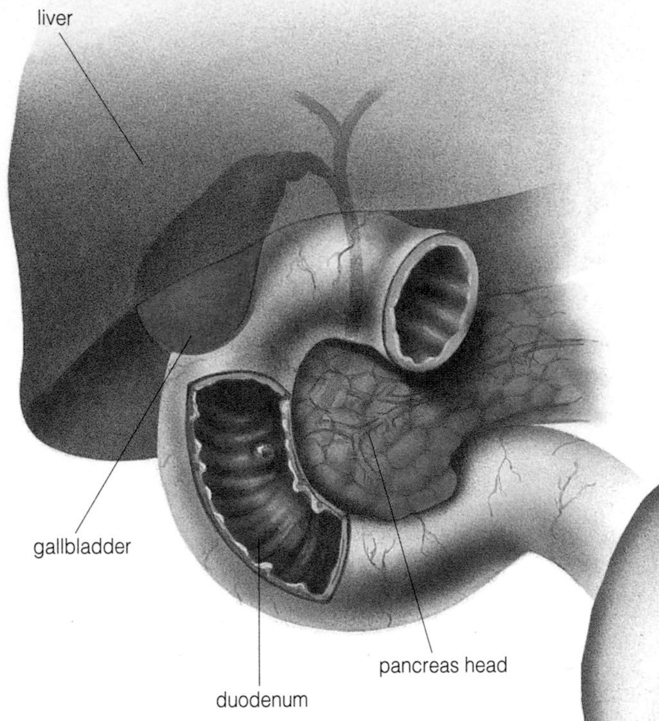

liver

gallbladder

duodenum

pancreas head

esophagus

liver

gallbladder

colon

stomach

colon

small intestine

rectum

anus

The stomach transforms solid foods into chyme, a thick liquid that passes slowly into the duodenum, the upper-most segment of the small intestine. There, most digestion takes place as bile and pancreatic enzymes and digestive juices go into action. After food is reduced to its basic molecules, it can be absorbed from the lining of the small intestine into the body.

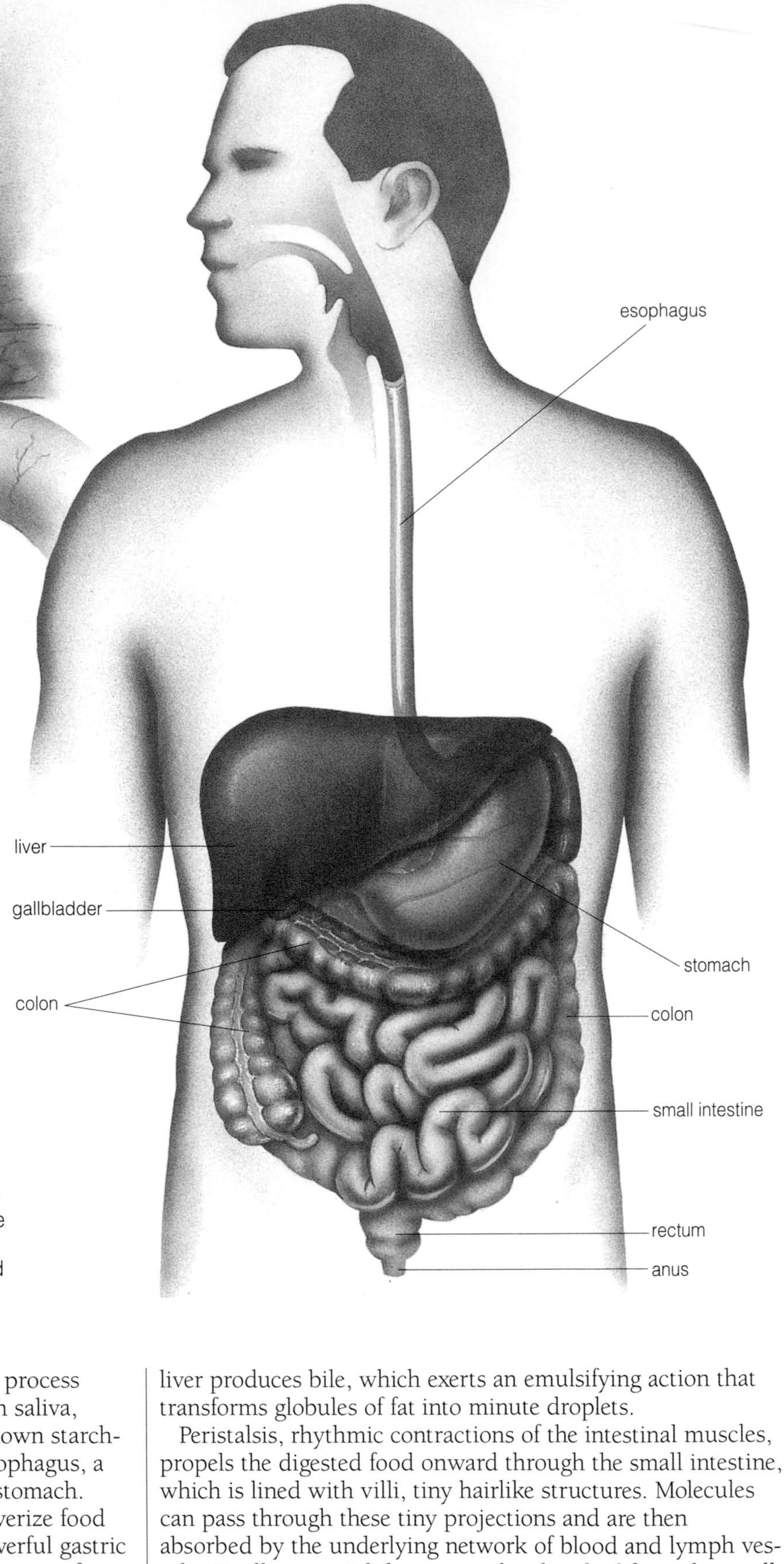

The human digestive system is comprised mostly of the alimentary canal, a 25-foot-long tube extending from the mouth to the anus. Most of this tube lies coiled in the abdominal cavity, where food is digested and absorbed and wastes are eliminated via the colon and rectum.

Digestion is a complex chemical and mechanical process that begins when food is chewed and mixed with saliva, which adds moisture and also begins breaking down starch-es. Swallowing forces a bolus of food into the esophagus, a 10-inch muscular tube that transports it to the stomach. Contractions of this muscular organ further pulverize food and mix it with hydrochloric acid and other powerful gastric juices. Little by little, the partially digested food passes from the stomach to the duodenum, the site of even more chemical action. Pancreatic enzymes and juices flow into this upper-most segment of the small intestine, where they break down proteins and carbohydrates. To make fats more soluble, the liver produces bile, which exerts an emulsifying action that transforms globules of fat into minute droplets.

Peristalsis, rhythmic contractions of the intestinal muscles, propels the digested food onward through the small intestine, which is lined with villi, tiny hairlike structures. Molecules can pass through these tiny projections and are then absorbed by the underlying network of blood and lymph ves-sels. Finally, material that cannot be absorbed from the small intestine passes into the colon. Here, fluid is extracted and returned to the circulation and the remaining fecal material is passed in a bowel movement. The total time required to fully digest a meal varies, but on average, it takes 24 to 36 hours.

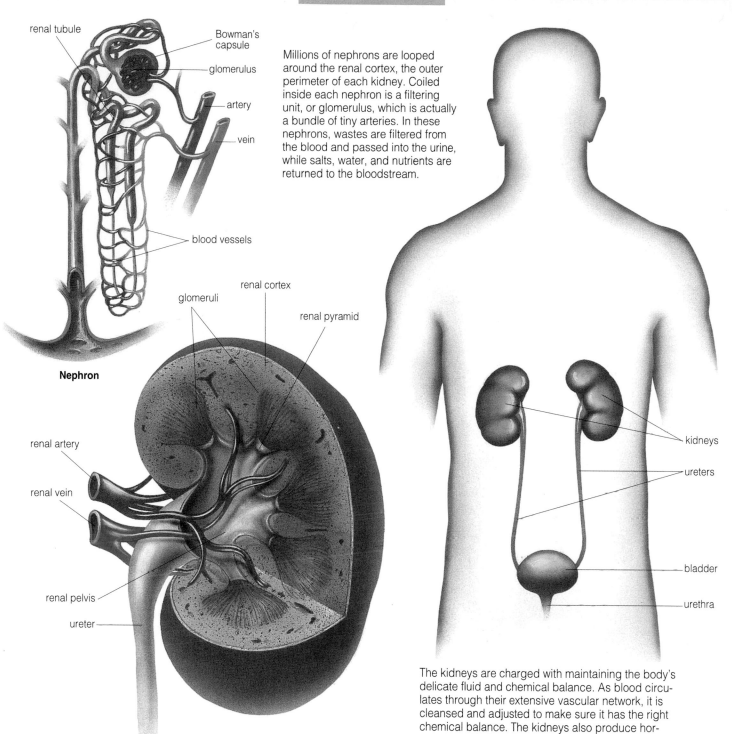

renal tubule

Bowman's capsule

glomerulus

artery

vein

blood vessels

Nephron

Millions of nephrons are looped around the renal cortex, the outer perimeter of each kidney. Coiled inside each nephron is a filtering unit, or glomerulus, which is actually a bundle of tiny arteries. In these nephrons, wastes are filtered from the blood and passed into the urine, while salts, water, and nutrients are returned to the bloodstream.

glomeruli

renal cortex

renal pyramid

renal artery

renal vein

renal pelvis

ureter

kidneys

ureters

bladder

urethra

The kidneys are charged with maintaining the body's delicate fluid and chemical balance. As blood circulates through their extensive vascular network, it is cleansed and adjusted to make sure it has the right chemical balance. The kidneys also produce hormones and help maintain blood pressure.

The body's excretory system is made up of a pair of kidneys and ureters, urinary bladder, and urethra. Kidneys do most of the work; the other structures transport or store urine.

The kidneys are bean-shaped organs, about four inches long and weighing only five ounces. They function as extraordinarily efficient chemical treatment plants, cleansing the blood of urea and other toxic wastes while maintaining the proper balance of fluid, salts, and other blood components. They are also instrumental in maintaining blood pressure.

The renal arteries branch off the abdominal aorta and carry a prodigious amount of blood. Each day, up to 500 quarts of fluid circulate through the kidneys. After it is cleansed, most of this fluid is returned to the bloodstream; only two to four pints are excreted as urine. This waste material collects in the central portion of the kidney—the renal pelvis—and from there it passes into the ureter, a long, narrow tube that carries the urine to the bladder. A normal adult bladder can hold about one pint of liquid, but when it is about half full, it begins to send nerve signals of an urge to urinate. Voluntary muscles in the pelvic floor control bladder function; when these muscles drop, the sphincter that controls the bladder opening relaxes and urine flows into the urethra. The female urethra is about 1.5 inches long and carries only urine; the 8-inch male urethra transports both semen and urine.

The respiratory system is often likened to an upside-down tree, with the trachea serving as the trunk, and the bronchi as the branches. The large bronchi branch out into ever smaller bronchioles, comparable to tree twigs.

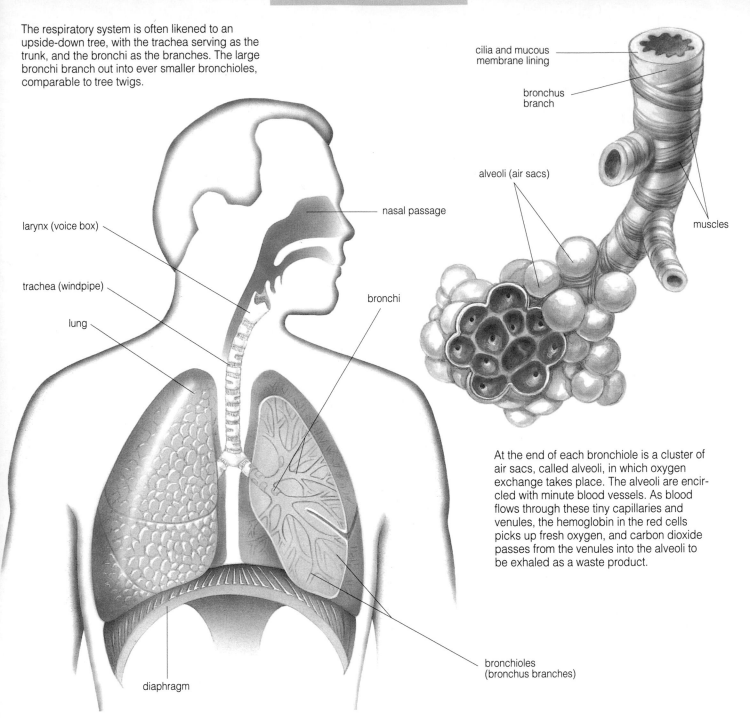

cilia and mucous membrane lining

bronchus branch

alveoli (air sacs)

muscles

larynx (voice box)

nasal passage

trachea (windpipe)

bronchi

lung

bronchioles (bronchus branches)

diaphragm

At the end of each bronchiole is a cluster of air sacs, called alveoli, in which oxygen exchange takes place. The alveoli are encircled with minute blood vessels. As blood flows through these tiny capillaries and venules, the hemoglobin in the red cells picks up fresh oxygen, and carbon dioxide passes from the venules into the alveoli to be exhaled as a waste product.

Of all the substances needed to sustain life, oxygen—an odorless, colorless, and tasteless gas—is perhaps the most critical because it is essential for all stages of metabolism, the various biochemical functions that maintain the body. Without oxygen, cells begin to die within minutes.

With each breath, oxygen is taken into the lungs and carbon dioxide and other wastes are expelled. Although you can deliberately hold your breath for a short period, breathing actually is an automatic process controlled by the brain's respiratory center. When performing quiet activities, a person takes about 14 breaths a minute, but the respiration rate may be slower during sleep or mediation and higher during exercise or other activities that demand extra oxygen.

Air is inhaled through the nose or mouth and passes through the larynx, or voice box, into the trachea, or the windpipe, and then to the bronchi and bronchioles, air tubes that branch off the trachea. These tubes are lined with millions of cilia, hairlike strands that beat rhythmically to keep dust, germs, and other airborne particles out of the lungs. The cilia also help clear the lungs of mucus produced by the mucous cells lining the bronchial tubes.

The bronchioles terminate in clusters of alveoli, tiny, balloon-like air sacs that are responsible for ensuring that the blood has a steady supply of fresh oxygen. Oxygen exchange takes place on the surface of the lungs' 700 million or so alveoli, which, if flattened out, would almost cover a tennis court. The air sacs are elastic, expanding during inhalation and deflating partially as air is exhaled. If alveoli lose their elasticity, as is the case in emphysema (page 175), stale air becomes trapped in the sacs and the body becomes starved for oxygen.

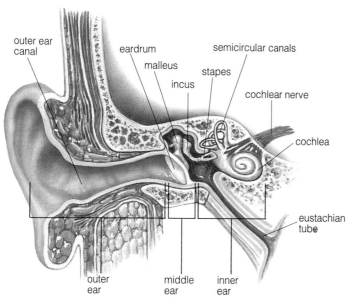

outer ear canal
eardrum
malleus
incus
stapes
semicircular canals
cochlear nerve
cochlea
eustachian tube
outer ear
middle ear
inner ear

eye muscle
sclera
choroid
iris
retina
cornea
anterior chamber (aqueous humor)
pupil
lens
ciliary body
optic nerve
vitreous chamber (vitreous humor)
eye muscle

Sound waves traveling through the air enter the outer ear and move through the middle ear into the inner ear, where they are transformed by an arrangement of tiny bones into vibrations. The vibrations then travel through fluid in the inner ear and are converted into electrical nerve impulses to be interpreted by the brain.

Light enters the eye through the lens and is focused on the retina at the back of the eyeball, where light-sensitive cells transform it into electrical impulses. The optic nerve then transmits these impulses to the brain, which interprets the image.

The tongue's surface is covered with millions of projections called papillae, giving it a furry, somewhat irregular surface. There are four types of papillae, three of which contain tastebuds. Although these buds can distinguish only four basic tastes—sour, sweet, salt, and bitter—complex nerve connections and the sense of smell allow us to detect subtle differences.

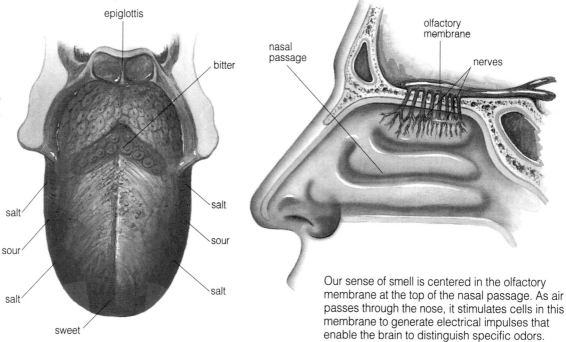

epiglottis
bitter
salt
salt
sour
sour
salt
salt
sweet

olfactory membrane
nasal passage
nerves

Our sense of smell is centered in the olfactory membrane at the top of the nasal passage. As air passes through the nose, it stimulates cells in this membrane to generate electrical impulses that enable the brain to distinguish specific odors.

Virtually everything that we perceive about our surroundings comes through information collected by the five basic senses—sight, hearing, taste, smell, and touch. Of these, sight and hearing are generally considered the most vital; in fact, however, all work in concert to provide a total picture. This cooperative process is especially apparent when you eat—odor is critical in distinguishing between foods that have a similar taste and texture. This is the reason that food seems to lack taste when you have a cold. However, when you are deprived of one particular sense, others can help compensate; for example, you can use touch and sound to find your way in the dark.

All sensory organs are complex extensions of the central nervous system (page 13), with a direct pathway to the brain, which allows instantaneous processing of information. (The eye's optic nerve is actually an extension of the brain.) The moment you touch an object, you know whether it is soft or hard, hot or cold, smooth or rough. Because information is processed so fast, we give little thought to the complexity of what is involved. Sounds entering the ear or light coming into the eye are immediately broken down and transformed into electrical impulses that are decoded and reassembled in the brain. A similar electrical transformation takes place in identifying an odor, interpreting a touch, and a recognizing a taste.

A finely tuned feedback system, directed by the hypothalamus in the brain, controls hormone levels throughout the body. The hypothalamus senses when levels of a certain hormone are low and passes this information on to the pituitary, which acts as the body's master gland. The pituitary immediately secretes hormones that signal another endocrine gland to pump out the needed hormone(s). When hormone levels are adequate, the hypothalamus switches off the pituitary's action.

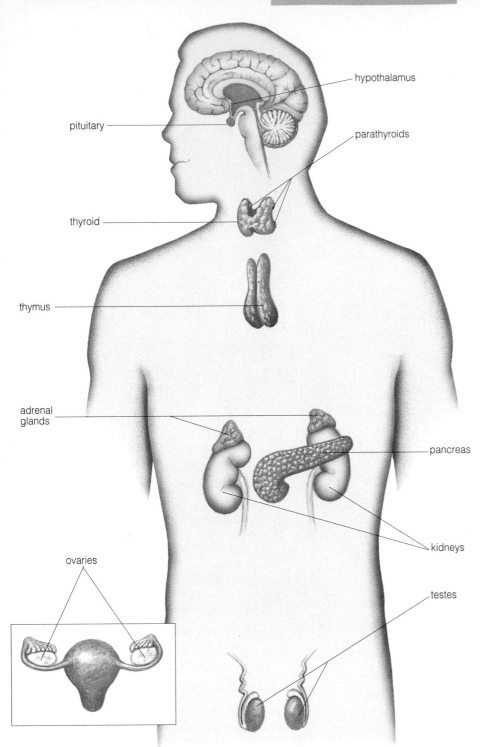

hypothalamus

pituitary

parathyroids

thyroid

thymus

adrenal glands

pancreas

kidneys

ovaries

testes

Each endocrine gland produces hormones that have specific functions throughout the body. Thyroid hormones, for example, control metabolism and are instrumental in normal growth and development. Calcitonin, also produced by the thyroid, lowers levels of calcium in the blood, while parathyroid hormones raise it. The thymus gland is instrumental in the immune system. Hormones produced by the adrenal glands trigger the body's fight-or-flight response to stress and also control levels of fluids and minerals and glucose metabolism. The pancreas makes insulin and glucagon, hormones that regulate blood levels of glucose. Finally, the gonads produce male and female sex hormones essential to reproduction.

Hormones are chemical messengers that influence virtually every body cell and function. Often working in concert with each other, as well as with the nervous system, hormones control growth, metabolism, digestion, blood pressure, reproduction, and response to stress, among many other functions. Understandably, hormonal imbalances can have profound effects throughout the body.

Although scientists know that hormones are key to almost every body process, much remains to be learned about how they work. For example, we still do not understand how the thymus and pineal glands and their hormones work. And from time to time, yet another hormone is discovered.

In addition to being produced by various endocrine glands, hormones are secreted by other organs, including the lungs, intestines, heart, and kidneys. Regardless of their origin, however, they all travel through the bloodstream in very small amounts, seeking out target organs or cells, which they then stimulate to perform a particular function. Some hormones, such as insulin, are too large to actually enter a cell; instead, they attach themselves to a preprogrammed receptor that triggers the desired response. Other hormones, such as the steroids produced by the adrenal glands, are small enough to penetrate target cells and elicit the desired response from its genetic material.

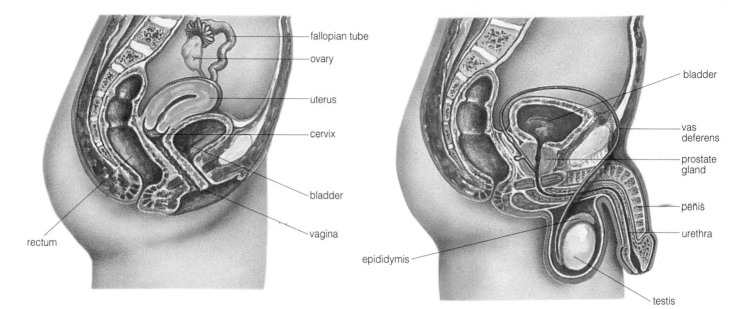

fallopian tube
ovary
uterus
cervix
bladder
vagina
rectum

bladder
vas deferens
prostate gland
penis
urethra
epididymis
testis

The female reproductive organs lie protected within the pelvic cavity, which can expand to accommodate a growing fetus. At birth, the ovaries harbor their lifetime complement of some 600,000 immature eggs, or oocytes. By puberty, many of these oocytes have disappeared; before menopause, about 400 will develop into mature ova; typically, one or two during a menstrual cycle.

The male reproductive system is designed to manufacture, store, and release sperm, beginning at puberty and continuing throughout life. An individual sperm takes an average of 72 days to mature, but huge numbers of sperm are constantly being made simultaneously; over a typical lifetime, a man produces some 12 trillion sperm.

Each month during a woman's reproductive years, an ovary is stimulated to mature a follicle, which then discharges a mature egg. The egg enters the fallopian tube where, if circumstances are right, fertilization takes place. Within 24 to 30 hours, the merged cell divides and over the next four days, it continues to divide as it travels to the uterus. In six to seven days, the embryo implants itself in the uterus lining, the endometrium, and continues to divide and grow. By the end of the first month, the fetus has begun to take shape, with a heart, budding arms and legs, and rudimentary eyes and central nervous system.

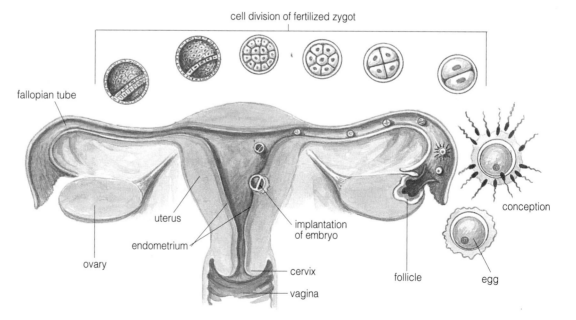

cell division of fertilized zygot
fallopian tube
uterus
endometrium
ovary
implantation of embryo
cervix
vagina
follicle
egg
conception

Reproduction remains one of life's most profound wonders. Just the notion that two barely visible cells can merge and form a new human being in just nine months is nothing short of a miracle. Of course, many things can go awry along the way, but most babies are healthy at birth with all the organs needed to grow into a normal adult.

Sex hormones—principally testosterone in men and estrogen in women—directly control reproduction. But many factors influence both the male and female reproductive systems, including overall health, nutrition, and stress. Genetics are also instrumental. Both the mother and father contribute half of the genes needed to make a new human being, and it is this genetic material that determines many of the offspring's characteristics, such as eye and hair color, height, body build, and blood type.

Sex is also determined at the moment of conception and depends upon which sex chromosome is donated by the father. Female cells have two X chromosomes; thus, when an egg divides, it must have an X chromosome. In contrast, males have an X and a Y chromosome, and a sperm can carry either one. So if an egg is fertilized by an X sperm, the baby will be a girl with two female X chromosomes; if the father contributes a Y sperm, the offspring will be a boy with the characteristic male XY chromosomes.

Most lymph nodes are clustered in the neck, armpits, abdomen, and groin. Fluid that drains from body tissues into the lymphatic system filters through at least one lymph node, where layers of tightly packed white blood cells attack and kill any harmful organisms. The swollen lymph nodes that are a sign of disease develop when large numbers of organisms or cancer cells collect in them.

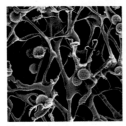

The above enlargement shows the internal filtering structure of a lymph node.

Blood vessels transport white blood cells, antibodies, and other protective substances produced by the immune system. The lymphatic system also returns body fluid to the bloodstream after it has been filtered through lymph nodes.

White blood cells are manufactured in the bone marrow and sent out into the blood-stream and lymphatic system. There are several types of white blood cells: Some are killer cells that destroy invading organisms, cancer cells, and other substances they recognize as foreign to body tissue; others release chemicals that cause inflammation, and still others engulf and digest bacteria.

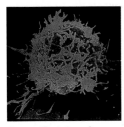

A magnified view of a T lymphocyte, a killer white blood cell.

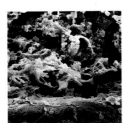

Developing red blood cells are seen as red dots in this enlarged view of bone marrow.

The tonsils are small masses of lymphoid tissue situated at the back of the throat. Along with the adenoids, these glands protect the upper respiratory tract against inhaled organisms. Unlike lymph nodes, the tonsils and adenoids are not enclosed in a capsule. Other clusters of nonencapsulated lymphoid tissue are located in parts of the small intestine.

The thymus is a gland made up of lymphoid tissue. White blood cells that pass through this gland are programmed to become T lymphocytes. The body's most abundant white blood cells, these protect against virus-es and other organisms. After puberty, the thymus gradually begins to shrink, although some active tissue remains into old age.

Lymph, a milky substance that con-tains white blood cells (lymphocytes), proteins, and fats, constantly bathes body tissues as it circulates through the network of lymphatic vessels. The lymphatic system does not have a pump like the heart; instead, lymph is kept moving through the vessels by movement of the body's muscles and a system of one-way valves.

The spleen, a fist-sized organ on the upper left side of the abdomen, is the body's largest lymph node. It has a dual function: As part of the immune system, it produces some antibod-ies and lymphocytes and helps filter and destroy invading organisms in the blood-stream; it also removes worn-out red blood cells from the bloodstream and breaks them down so that their iron can be reused. Despite its importance, the spleen is not an essential organ; if it must be removed due to injury or disease, its immune system functions are assumed by other lymphatic tissue.

The human body is constantly bombarded by millions of viruses, bacteria, and other disease-causing microorganisms, or pathogens. Fortunately, most of these are thwarted by the body's own protective physical and chemical barriers, such as the skin, saliva, tears, mucus, and stomach acid. The mil-lions of bacteria that live on the skin and the body's mucous membranes also help protect against certain invaders. When a pathogen does manage to evade these defenses and enter the body, it is attacked almost immediately by one or more components of the immune system.

The immune system uses extremely sensitive chemical sen-sors to recognize a foreign organism or tissue, especially one that can cause disease. Sometimes it overreacts to a harmless substance, such as pollen or a certain food or medication; this can set the stage for an allergic reaction. In other cases, the immune system mistakenly attacks normal body tissue as if it were foreign, resulting in an autoimmune disease such as lupus or rheumatoid arthritis. Most of the time, however, the immune system holds fast as our first line of defense against a host of potentially deadly diseases.

Infectious Agents

Disease-causing organisms vary from tiny viruses to parasites such as the tapeworm, which can grow 20 feet long. Regardless of the size or species of the invading organism, a healthy immune system will mount a vigorous defense against it. The exact nature of that defense varies, however, according to the type and number of invading organisms. The more common types are illustrated below.

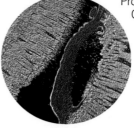

Protozoa are tiny single-celled organisms. Common protozoal infections include giardiasis, an intestinal infection caused by drinking giardia-infected water, and toxoplasmosis, which comes from eating undercooked meat or handling the feces of an infected cat.

Bacteria come in many shapes, including the spheres of various cocci species (staphylococci is shown below), the rods of bacilli, and the spirals of spirochetes like those that cause Lyme disease and syphilis.

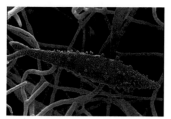

Viruses, the smallest and most prevalent of all life forms, can multiply only after invading the cell of another organism. The enlargement below shows the hepatitis B virus.

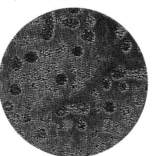

Fungi are yeast-like parasites that most commonly grow on the skin or mucous membranes. Ringworm of the scalp is shown above; other common fungal infections include yeast vaginitis and athlete's foot.

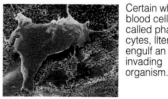

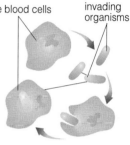

Various worms, or helminths, such as roundworms (left), are parasites that cause diseases.

How the Immune System Fights Infection

Whenever a foreign organism enters the body, chemical signals send the immune system into action. Different types of white blood cells rush to the site of infection to halt the organisms from spreading to other parts of the body.

Organisms that manage to escape the body's first line of defense are met with more concerted and complicated efforts. One calls into action B lymphocytes, white cells that are programmed to recognize a specific organism. In the presence of this organism, the B cells multiply rapidly, producing memory cells that can change into plasma cells; the latter then make antibodies to seek out and destroy the organism. After the infection, remaining memory cells are prepared to go into action if again confronted with the same disease organism.

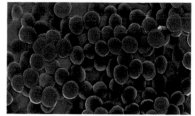

Certain white blood cells, called phagocytes, literally engulf an invading organism.

As part of the immune system's first line of defense, killer lymphocytes release chemicals to destroy invading organisms, while mast cells and eosinophils release substances that produce inflammation. If the invader is a virus, specialized white cells give off interferons, proteins that prevent viruses from reproducing in body cells.

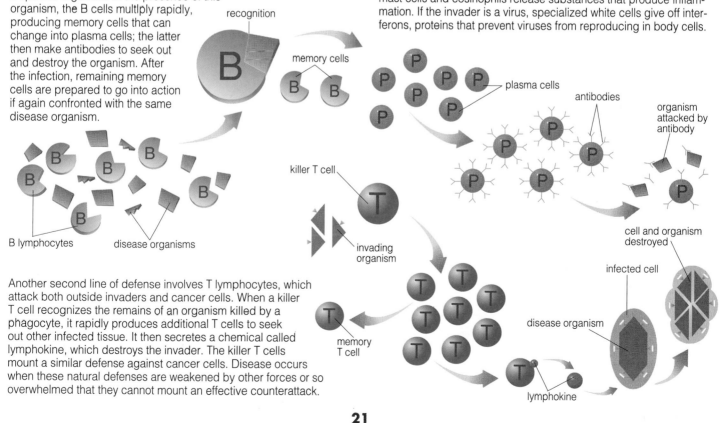

B lymphocytes

disease organisms

recognition

memory cells

plasma cells

antibodies

organism attacked by antibody

killer T cell

invading organism

memory T cell

lymphokine

disease organism

infected cell

cell and organism destroyed

white blood cells

invading organisms

Another second line of defense involves T lymphocytes, which attack both outside invaders and cancer cells. When a killer T cell recognizes the remains of an organism killed by a phagocyte, it rapidly produces additional T cells to seek out other infected tissue. It then secretes a chemical called lymphokine, which destroys the invader. The killer T cells mount a similar defense against cancer cells. Disease occurs when these natural defenses are weakened by other forces or so overwhelmed that they cannot mount an effective counterattack.

New Choices in Healing

Medicine is undergoing a quiet revolution. Only a few years ago, most mainstream physicians and practitioners of alternative therapies tended to view each other with suspicion, if not disdain. Physicians often charged that alternative practitioners were charlatans; in turn, therapists outside of the mainstream claimed that doctors relied too much on potentially dangerous drugs and surgery, and were so overly specialized that they failed to treat the patient as a whole.

Increasingly, both camps are recognizing that each has a place in the healing process—a trend that is being embraced by a growing number of patients. For example, at least one-third of respondents in a 1990 survey said that they had been to alternative practitioners. Most patients also saw physicians, but the researchers estimated that visits to alternative practitioners actually exceeded those to primary-care physicians. In keeping with the trend, some insurance policies now cover certain alternative therapies, especially if the treatments are recommended by a physician.

The Historic Perspective

Until the early part of the 20th century, physicians and alternative practitioners competed more or less on equal footing in North America, because there were few standards or regulations. Thus, the traveling medicine man could legally call himself a doctor and peddle worthless patent medicines.

This changed dramatically in 1910, when strict standards, based on scientific principles, were adopted for medical schools in Canada and the United States. Within a few years, only graduates from accredited medical schools could practice medicine, and homeopathy, chiropractic, and other "unorthodox" disciplines were shunned by the medical profession. If the benefits of a therapy could not be documented scientifically, it was discounted as worthless. Some, such as homeopathy, virtually disappeared, and others, such as chiropractic, were relegated to a questionable gray area. Of course, real quackery did not disappear, but government agencies and regulations made life more difficult for charlatans as well as for legitimate alternative practitioners.

Searching for a Common Ground

The pendulum began to swing back with the development of osteopathy and psychiatry as recognized medical specialties, and acceptance of the ancient observation that emotional factors play an important role in health and illness. The 1960s brought renewed interest in Eastern philosophy and healing practices, as well as growing polarization between scientific medicine and alternative therapies. Still, it became increasingly difficult for physicians to discount benefits of certain alternative practices, and conventional medicine started to embrace some of them. In particular, pain clinics began to incorporate such therapies as acupuncture, meditation, and biofeedback training into their therapeutic regimens.

As college graduates of the sixties matured and some entered medical school, a middle ground began to emerge between the two opposing groups. There are still diehards at each extreme, but their numbers are decreasing as more physicians and alternative practitioners recognize that neither has all of the answers but both have things to offer. The basic principles and modalities of conventional medicine are discussed on pages 24–31; while natural, or alternative, therapies are covered on pages 32–61.

A Medical System in Transition

A few decades ago, most families relied upon a general practitioner to look after most of their medical needs. This doctor delivered babies, treated childhood illnesses, set broken bones, performed surgery, and comforted the aged and dying. But lacking vaccines, antibiotics, and other modern medications and daring surgical procedures, these doctors were helpless against many of the serious diseases that are now easily cured.

Today, with the growing complexity of conventional medicine, more doctors are specializing in specific parts of the body. Consequently, families are likely to be attended by several doctors. Faced with a rapidly changing health care system, skyrocketing health-care costs, and so many medical specialists and subspecialists, patients may feel uncertain about where to start when they have medical problems. They are baffled by the technology and complexity of modern medicine, and may feel alienated from their physicians, who perhaps don't take the time to explain various procedures.

Experts agree that it's essential in this era of medical specialization for individuals to have a primary physician to oversee and coordinate care. Most primary-care physicians are trained in family practice, internal medicine, pediatrics, or gynecology. If you have a chronic disorder such as heart disease, diabetes, arthritis, or other serious health problem, your primary doctor may specialize in that area, and still oversee your care for other problems. Whenever sickness strikes, you should start by seeing your primary doctor, who can, if appropriate, refer you to specialists.

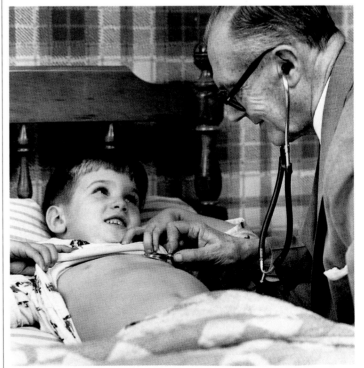

Gone are the days when a family doctor was expected to make routine house calls and treat family members of all ages for a wide range of ailments.

The Diagnostic Process

All medical treatment hinges on an accurate diagnosis, and this begins with a careful medical history. Often, your doctor can zero in on what's ailing you simply by asking the right questions. Of course, you must describe your concerns and symptoms truthfully and accurately. Patients are sometimes afraid to bring up what's really worrying them, and they wait for the doctor to broach the subject. On the other hand, talking about deeply personal matters, even to a doctor, can be embarrassing. It's important to be as forthcoming as possible.

After taking a medical history, the doctor does a physical examination. Although the emphasis varies according to the symptoms, a typical exam usually includes measuring your height, weight, and blood pressure, and checking your heart and other organs, abdomen, mouth, throat, and eyes for any abnormalities. Routine laboratory tests—blood and urine analyses and perhaps a chest X-ray and an electrocardiogram (ECG)—round out a complete physical. If more information is needed, additional tests may be ordered, or a medical specialist consulted. After gathering as much data as possible, the doctor interprets it and arrives at a diagnosis.

NEW INSIGHTS INTO THE HUMAN BODY

New imaging techniques allow doctors to examine virtually every internal organ without resorting to exploratory surgery. In addition to standard X-rays, these include the following:

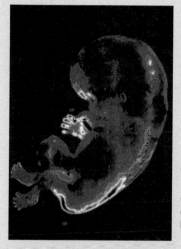

▶ Ultrasound, in which high-frequency sound waves are used in a system similar to sonar for producing images. The waves enter the body painlessly and reflect off internal organs. These reflections can be seen on a video monitor; a computer also records the patterns of reflection and prints out images for later analysis. An audio component can be added to study blood flow through various vessels. Ultrasound is especially useful during pregnancy, because it does not expose the fetus to harmful X-rays or drugs.

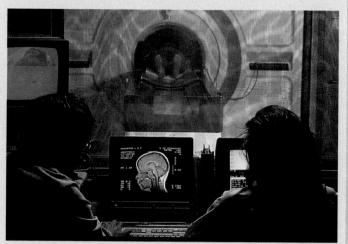

▶ Magnetic resonance imaging, or MRI, in which a powerful magnet instead of the radiation of an X-ray produces three-dimensional views of internal organs. The technique is based on the physics principle that every atom in the body has a nucleus. Radio waves from the MRI machine's magnet, directed into the body, temporarily move the nuclei out of alignment. When the radio waves are stopped, the nuclei move back to their normal alignment, creating signals that are transmitted to a computer and converted into three-dimensional video and film images.

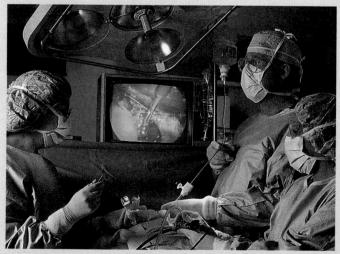

▶ Fiberoptics, in which powerful lights and magnifying devices allow doctors to view internal organs directly. The fiberoptic devices are contained in thin tubes, or catheters, that are inserted into the body through the mouth, anus, or other natural opening, or via a small incision. Common fiberoptic examinations include colonoscopy to study the large intestine, laparoscopy to examine the abdominal cavity, and arthoscopy to view the inside of a joint. During the examination, tissue samples can be collected. Also, many operations, such as removal of colon polyps or repair of a joint, can be performed using fiberoptic technology.

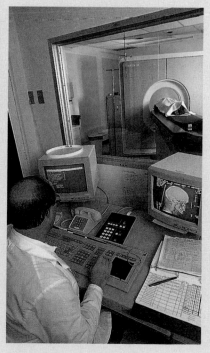

▶ Computed tomography, or CT scans, in which multiple X-rays create a three-dimensional view of a cross-section of the body. The patient is placed inside a scanning machine, while an X-ray unit takes hundreds of films as it revolves around the part of the body under examination. A computer reconstructs the multiple images into a three-dimensional view of a cross section of the body. To make organs stand out, a contrast dye may be used. Color can also be added to the images.

Conventional Medicine

Conventional, or allopathic, medicine focuses mostly on the diagnosis and treatment of disease, although preventive practices as part of this system have gained considerable influence in recent years.

Obviously, treatments vary according to the disorder, but all are aimed at reversing or repairing the underlying condition. If a cure is impossible, the doctor tries to manage or ease the symptoms as much as possible.

Before prescribing a specific course of treatment, a physician weighs the potential benefits against the possible risks. Sometimes the risks or costs of treatment outweigh possible benefits; in other cases, the condition may not warrant immediate treatment but require periodic monitoring. In any event, you as the patient should participate as an informed partner with your doctor in all decision making.

Types of Treatment

All conventional treatments are classified in one of three categories: preventive, noninvasive, or surgery (invasive).

Preventive medicine emphasizes taking specific action to forestall disease. Some aspects are so commonplace that we take them for granted. For example, many killer diseases of the past are now rare or, in the case of smallpox, extinct, thanks to routine immunization. Improved sanitation and other public health measures have rendered cholera, plague, and typhoid fever rare in industrialized nations, but they are still rampant in undeveloped countries and, given the right circumstances, can spread to developed nations.

Often, preventive medicine calls for a wait-and-see approach in which patients have frequent checkups, but no specific therapy is prescribed. For example, if your family medical history indicates that you have a high risk of developing cancer of the breast or the colon, you will probably be advised to undergo regular screening examinations to look for any suspicious changes. This allows your doctor to detect cancer in its earliest, most treatable stage.

In other cases, the preventive measures might include drug therapy or even surgery. For instance, low-dose aspirin and other drugs are prescribed routinely now to prevent a heart attack in a high-risk patient. Some people who have a hereditary type of colon polyps that invariably develop into colon cancer may be advised to have a preventive colectomy, an operation in which the entire colon is removed.

Most often, however, preventive medicine emphasizes a healthy lifestyle. Experts now agree that our most common killer diseases can often be prevented by not smoking, by exercising regularly, eating a well-balanced diet, maintaining normal weight, and controlling stress. For many people, certain aspects of alternative medicine, such as meditation, yoga, massage, and biofeedback, have become an important part of their preventive regimens.

Noninvasive therapy, usually entails taking drugs, ranging from an occasional nonprescription painkiller to an intensive regimen of chemotherapy for cancer. (Other noninvasive modalities include radiation, sound waves, and psychological counseling.) The introduction of scores of new drugs in the last 50 years has forever changed the practice of medicine. At the turn of the century, infectious diseases were the leading cause of death, and the average life expectancy was about 50 years. Today, not only do vaccines prevent many diseases that formerly killed people in their youth, but antibiotics can also cure most bacterial infections. Consequently, life expectancy in Canada now exceeds 77 years.

Serious incurable diseases such as diabetes and high blood pressure can be controlled by drugs. Similarly, drugs help minimize the crippling effects of arthritis and control many forms of mental illness. But much remains to be done. AIDS and other deadly diseases still defy a cure; researchers hope that these will soon be conquered by drugs or vaccines.

Although drugs can be life-saving, they can also produce adverse side effects that range from minor and annoying to potentially fatal. Medications are not "magic bullets" that attack only the disease; instead, they affect the entire body. Some trigger the immune system to mount an allergic reaction; others damage healthy as well as diseased tissue; and still others produce quite unpredictable reactions. A few of the latter have led to new drug uses and discoveries. For example, the observation that certain allergy medications reduce appetite resulted in the development of new diet pills; the ability of a blood pressure drug to stimulate hair growth produced a somewhat effective treatment for baldness.

Researchers are always seeking to minimize any adverse side effects by devising new ways to deliver medications to their target tissues and bypass organs that would be adversely affected. Some of these are already in use. For example, medicated skin patches effectively deliver small, steady amounts of drugs directly into the bloodstream, thus avoiding the potential problems of having larger doses circulating at any time.

A healthy lifestyle, which includes a nutritious diet, plenty of exercise, and control of weight and stress, is the best preventive medicine.

Enteric coatings that cause a pill to remain intact until it reaches the small intestine protect the stomach from irritation. Cloning techniques that produce special antibodies to carry drugs make it easier to target cancer drugs on tumor cells while sparing normal tissue.

Fetuses, young children, and the elderly are especially vulnerable to adverse drug effects, and in these groups, medications should be used only under a doctor's careful supervision. In general, medicines must always be used cautiously, if at all, during pregnancy, and dosages should be carefully adjusted for children and the elderly.

For anyone, the risk of adverse drug effects increases with the number of medications taken simultaneously because many drugs interact with each other. These dangers can be minimized by always giving a doctor and pharmacist a list of all medications you are taking—including vitamins and non-prescription drugs—before adding more. Many pharmacists now keep computer patient drug profiles, making it easy to spot potentially harmful combinations.

Surgery, an invasive procedure that requires making an incision and using various instruments to enter the body, has also made tremendous advances in recent years. It is an ancient art that was typically practiced in years past by barbers and veterinarians, rather than physicians. Until the 20th century, surgery had a high mortality rate from infection and other complications. Modern anesthesia and antiseptic techniques revolutionized the practice, making most operations painless with greatly reduced risk.

There are now hundreds of different surgical procedures. Operations are performed to repair a damaged structure, to remove a diseased organ, or to alleviate a chronic symptom such as pain. In some instances, surgery may be aimed at preventing a future disease or problem; such a case would be removal of a benign growth to prevent its becoming cancerous. Some operations, especially cosmetic plastic surgery, are intended primarily to enhance self-esteem and a sense of well-being rather than alleviate a medical problem. Doctors may also use surgical procedures, such as biopsies and exploratory surgery, to help in making a diagnosis.

In the 1970s and 1980s, surgery underwent another revolution: Development of powerful surgical microscopes and fiberoptic techniques made it possible to perform delicate operations through tiny puncture incisions. For example, some back surgery that once required a long incision and weeks of recuperation can now be performed using microsurgery methods that necessitate only a brief hospital stay.

Coronary bypass surgery and other heart operations that were impossible a few decades ago are now routine. In fact, critics charge that a large percentage of bypass procedures are unnecessary, and that many patients would do just as well with medication and lifestyle changes. In nonemergency cases many insurance companies and other third-party payers now require a presurgery second opinion to make sure that the operation is really needed. (See box, lower left.)

For some diseases, most notably cancer, surgery is the major treatment. But it is often combined with other approaches, such as radiation and chemotherapy, to produce even better results. Similarly, arthritis treatment may entail a combination of medication and exercise, as well as surgery.

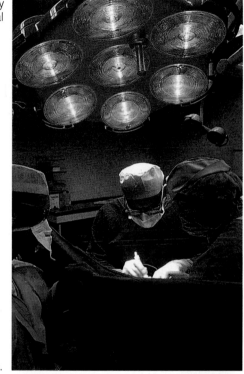

Fiberoptic technology and powerful surgical microscopes now enable surgeons to perform complex procedures through tubes inserted into tiny incisions or natural body openings.

Small amounts of powerful chemotherapy drugs for cancer are often combined to increase their effectiveness and minimize side effects.

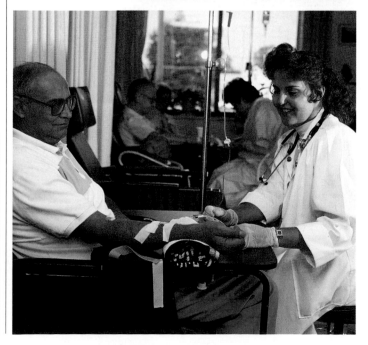

SHOULD YOU SEEK A SECOND OPINION?

Although there have been tremendous advances in modern surgical techniques, it is advisable to make sure that an operation is the best treatment option. In particular, always seek a second opinion before having any of the following operations:

Cataract removal	Knee surgery
Coronary artery bypass and other heart operations	Prostate surgery
Gallbladder removal	Spinal disk removal and other back operations
Hernia repair	
Hysterectomy	Tonsillectomy

Laboratory Medicine

Once doctors had to depend exclusively on their own observations and on the patient's description of symptoms to diagnose a disease and monitor treatment. Today, all doctors rely on laboratory tests in making their decisions. Some of these tests may be done on samples of blood, urine, or body tissue. For others, the patient may be sent to a special laboratory for X-rays (page 27), function studies (described below), or scans, imaging, or certain invasive procedures such as colonoscopy (explained on page 23). The type of tests you'll be given often depends on your age, health, personal and family history, as well as your doctor's preferences. The following are some of the most common tests that you may encounter as part of a diagnostic process. If they reveal a potential health problem, more complex testing may be required:

Urinalysis. Urine studies are the oldest medical tests. Ancient physicians diagnosed disease by studying the color

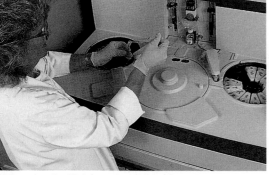

Modern medical laboratories are equipped with a wide array of sophisticated machines that can perform multiple tests using a single blood sample.

and smell of urine, and some even tasted it. By this last method, early Greek physicians could discern diabetes, when the urine had a sweet taste because of the presence of blood sugar, or glucose. Today, urine is studied not only for glucose, but also for blood cells, protein, bacteria, hormones, and chemicals. Some urine tests can be done at home. Included are early pregnancy tests, which can now detect pregnancy as soon as two weeks after conception; and a glucose test, in which chemical strips dipped in a urine sample can detect sugar, a sign that diabetes is out of control. For other analyses, the urine specimen may be collected at home or in a doctor's office, and then sent to a laboratory.

Blood tests. Your blood speaks volumes about your health, and blood tests can detect many conditions long before any symptoms appear. Certain of these tests involve measuring levels of substances carried in the blood, such as cholesterol, hormones, enzymes, drugs, and numerous body chemicals. A biochemical profile, which may involve 40 or more such measurements, can now be done very quickly in a sequential multiple analyzer (SMA) machine. The results of your blood test are reported on a computer printout that compares your numbers with the normal ones.

Although automated blood analysis is fast and relatively inexpensive, errors are common, and you should not be unduly alarmed by an abnormal result. In such cases, a

second, less automated, and more precise test will be done to confirm the results of the first one.

Other tests involve looking through a microscope at the blood cells themselves. For a total blood count, the numbers of different blood cells in a specific amount of blood are estimated. The size, shapes, and color of the cells may also be studied, especially if sickle cell disease, anemia, leukemia, or another type of blood disorder is suspected.

Biopsies. These tests require examination of a sample of tissue under a microscope for abnormalities. In some biopsies, a tumor or piece of tissue is removed surgically. In other cases, such as in a bone, liver, or breast biopsy, the sample may be obtained by aspiration with a hollow needle inserted through the skin and overlying tissue.

Pap smear. This test involves scraping cells from the surface of a woman's cervix and then studying them microscopically for abnormalities that may indicate the possibility of cancer. Pap smears, which are included as part of most gynecological examinations, should be performed every one to three years. The test is not painful and usually lasts only about five minutes.

Function tests. These are diagnostic studies done in special laboratories to assess how well an organ or organ system is functioning. Common examples include hearing and vision tests, spirometry to assess lung function, exercise stress tests to study cardiovascular capability, and nerve and muscle studies. In some cases, such as a fertility work-up, function tests are usually combined with other types of laboratory analyses.

The Effectiveness of Testing

In recent years, laboratory testing has emerged as one of the the fastest growing aspects of medical care. Computers and other technological advances are responsible for much of this growth. In some cases, screening tests only rarely reveal abnormality, raising questions about their effectiveness. For example, ultrasound is now performed frequently during pregnancy to screen for certain birth defects and determine fetal age. Some health experts question whether this is an appropriate use of medical resources because the large majority of pregnancies are normal. As an alternative, they suggest that ultrasound be reserved for high-risk pregnancies or those in which a problem is already suspected.

Moreover, many tests are highly uncomfortable and some carry a risk of complications. As a patient, you can protect yourself from being given any unnecessary tests by asking the following questions:

▶ Why do I need this test?
▶ Is it painful?
▶ Is there any risk of complications?
▶ How accurate, usually, are the results?
▶ Am I likely to need additional tests?
▶ How will the results be used?
▶ Will the results affect the course of my treatment?
▶ What will happen if I don't have the test?

Nuclear Medicine

Nuclear medicine involves the use of radioactive materials for either diagnosis or treatment. Until the 1950s, the technology was confined to diagnostic X-rays and radiation treatments for cancer and a few other diseases. Today, it is used in the most sophisticated diagnostic studies and surgical procedures, and includes such subspecialties as nuclear cardiology.

For diagnostic X-rays, relatively low doses of ionizing radiation are beamed through soft tissue onto photographic film, where they make denser tissue, such as bone, stand out.

For therapy, radiation is given in larger doses that kill body tissues by destroying the ability of cells to grow and divide normally. It is especially lethal to tissue that grows fast, with a rapid rate of renewal. This is why it is effective in shrinking and eventually eliminating cancerous tumors. Today, half of all cancer patients receive some form of radiation therapy.

Because radiation cannot distinguish between cancerous and normal tissue, it also damages healthy cells, particularly in the skin, the linings of many internal organs, and the bone marrow, where blood cells are made. If the radiation dosage is not too high, most normal tissue will eventually repair itself. Thus, the challenge is to find a dosage that will kill a cancer without rendering permanent damage to the healthy surrounding tissue. Complicating matters is the fact that radiation damage is cumulative. Even low-level environmental, or background, radiation contributes to the buildup.

The Newer Technologies

As medical researchers learn more about the harmful effects of radiation, they are developing ever safer ways to use it. New technology allows doctors to implant tiny radioactive seeds in some types of tumors to shrink or destroy them while sparing healthy tissue. This approach is now being used for prostate cancer and certain inoperable tumors.

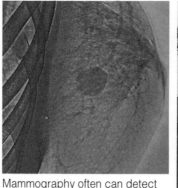
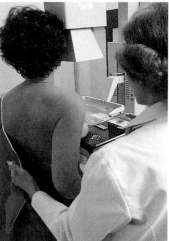

Mammography often can detect breast cancers that are too small to be felt during a physical examination. Above is a mammogram showing a small tumor.

In treating other cancerous growths, computers enable therapists to calculate the precise dosage required and new machines beam radiation directly to the tumor. In still other instances, chemicals carry radiation to an organ without exposing other parts of the body. For example, the use of radioactive iodine often removes the need for surgery in the treatment of an overactive thyroid gland; the thyroid absorbs the iodine, and the radiation destroys part or all of the gland's hormone-making tissue.

New X-ray equipment also delivers less radiation than in the past. The newest mammography machines, for example, require less than one-third of the amount of radiation needed only 20 years ago. In addition, the injection of minute amounts of radioactive particles that can be followed by special gamma cameras allows doctors to study internal organs with less radiation and more accuracy than is possible with X-ray machines alone. For instance, a radioactive material called thallium is used in making heart scans that pinpoint areas where the cardiac muscle is not getting enough blood.

Despite the tremendous advances in nuclear medicine, it is important to realize that there is still a risk involved in exposure to any radiation. Avoid routine diagnostic X-rays unless their benefit clearly outweighs the risk. Hence, the potential risk of an annual chest X-ray is greater than the possible benefits for a healthy person. In contrast, mammography every one or two years for women over the age of 50 is currently recommended because the risk of breast cancer is much higher than any known hazards of this X-ray examination.

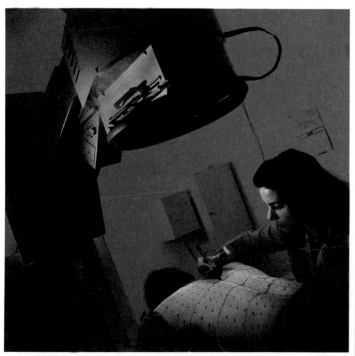

Powerful X-ray machines can be programmed to deliver large amounts of tumor-killing radiation to a very small area, thus sparing as much normal tissue as possible.

RADIATION AND BIRTH DEFECTS

X-rays and other forms of ionizing radiation are especially harmful to a developing fetus; they can cause severe birth defects or even fetal death. Any woman who is pregnant, or who may be pregnant without knowing it, should not be X-rayed. If an X-ray is absolutely necessary, a protective lead shield should be used to cover the fetus.

Even before conception, radiation can cause birth defects by damaging the father's sperm or the mother's eggs. With time, a man's ability to produce healthy sperm usually returns. But a woman does not make new eggs; she is born with her lifetime supply. Fortunately, surgical techniques now allow the ovaries to be moved out of the field of exposure during radiation therapy, and later returned to their normal position.

Psychiatry and Psychotherapy

At some point, one out of every three North Americans suffers a mental disorder serious enough to benefit from treatment. Unfortunately, among those who need therapy, only 20 to 25 percent of adults and 60 percent of children undergo it. Why is mental illness so neglected? Experts note that even in this enlightened age, it still carries a social stigma, and large numbers of people who could be helped elect to suffer in silence. Others try to heal themselves, often with little or no success. Still others recognize that they have a problem, but don't know where to go for help, or cannot afford the usually high cost of therapy (see box, below).

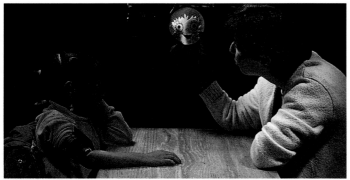

Puppets can allow troubled children to express feelings and concerns they may consider too shameful or frightening to discuss openly.

An Expanding Field

At one time, psychiatry dealt mostly with severe and incapacitating mental illness. Today, psychiatrists and other mental health professionals are called upon to treat a wide range of problems: eating disorders, sexual dysfunction, marital problems, stress-related diseases, personality problems, violent and aggressive behavior, alcoholism and substance abuse, and sleep disorders, among others. As with other medical specialties, mental health professionals tend to concentrate on one or two areas; it might be family therapy, for example, child psychiatry, or treatment of mood disorders.

Psychoactive Drugs

Treatment of mental illness has changed dramatically since the 1950s, when psychoactive drugs were first introduced (see box, opposite page). Before, patients with severe mental illness were institutionalized. Now potent tranquilizers and other drugs enable them to live independently, or at least outside of a mental hospital. Although millions of people have been helped by these new drugs, there are drawbacks. For

GUIDE TO MENTAL HEALTH PROFESSIONALS

TITLE	WHO THEY ARE AND WHAT THEY DO
Psychiatrists	diagnose and treat mental disorders that are either organic or psychological in origin. Because they are physicians, they can also prescribe drugs.
Clinical psychologists	treat psychological, behavior, and personality disorders. Most have doctorate degrees in psychology and can do psychotherapy, but cannot prescribe drugs or treat any organic illness.
Psychiatric social workers	specialize in counseling patients with mental or emotional problems. They often team up with psychiatrists.
Psychiatric nurses	work in a hospital or mental health clinic, with a psychiatrist, or in private practice. They are registered nurses who have advanced training in treating patients with mental illness.
Counselors	give counsel to distressed persons. In most states, there are no legal definitions or requirements for such personnel. Some have formal training, others are self-styled, and still others are members of the clergy or related professions.

the most part, they do not cure, but instead help to bring the disease under control—a process that usually requires continuing therapy. In treating manic-depression and schizophrenia, for example, life-long drug therapy is necessary, usually in conjunction with counseling.

Persons undergoing this combined approach can often lead productive, relatively normal lives, especially in group homes or similar settings. Too often, however, they are left on their own and may relapse after stopping medication. Mental health experts estimate that more than one-third of the homeless people in North American cities are patients who would have been institutionalized in the past.

Side effects of psychoactive drugs pose other hazards, which range from drowsiness and movement disorders to addiction and fatal overdoses. Finding the right dosage or combination of drugs to minimize such effects can be costly and time-consuming. And psychoactive drugs must always be used under close medical supervision.

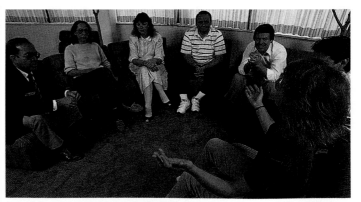

Group psychotherapy is a less expensive alternative to individual therapy. It can also be an adjunct to one-on-one psychotherapy or inpatient treatment, particularly for substance abuse.

LOW-COST ALTERNATIVES

One-on-one psychotherapy is an expensive, long-term undertaking. Some insurance policies cover psychotherapy, but most limit their coverage. Short-term goal-oriented therapy, which is less costly, is covered by most insurance plans. Other low-cost alternatives include group therapy (right), mental health clinics, and counseling provided by psychiatric social workers.

Nondrug Therapies

Even if psychoactive drugs are prescribed, nondrug therapy is also recommended. The type of approach varies according to the underlying illness, and may include the following:

Psychodynamic psychotherapy attempts to uncover the source of mental disturbance by having the patient talk freely, especially about childhood experiences and dreams. In its classic Freudian form, it is conducted individually, with the patient talking while the therapist listens. One-on-one psychoanalysis is the most intensive, lengthy, and expensive form of psychotherapy, requiring from one to five sessions a week for three to five years. Variations on this approach include group, couple, or family therapy, in which a therapist treats more than one patient simultaneously.

Short or time-limited psychotherapy has evolved as a popular alternative to classic psychotherapy. In this approach, the patient and therapist agree upon a specific goal and the number of sessions needed to achieve it.

Cognitive therapy, which is also a short-term treatment, seeks to identify and correct distorted thought processes that result in self-defeating behavior. For example, if you are invariably late in meeting assignments because you cannot get started before a deadline looms, the therapist will help pinpoint the attitudes responsible for your poor work habits, and suggest ways to change them. This approach is especially effective in treating depression.

Behavior modification focuses on correcting a faulty habit or behavior without addressing any of the underlying psychological aspects. It is especially helpful in overcoming phobias, bad habits such as smoking, eating disorders, and certain compulsive behavior such as obsessive hand-washing.

ELECTROCONVULSIVE THERAPY

Electroconvulsive therapy (ECT) is a controversial and much misunderstood treatment for severe mental illness. During this process, pulses of electrical current are administered to the brain, producing brief seizures. Doctors do not fully understand how it works, but ECT remains one of the most effective treatments for severe suicidal depression. It is also recommended for psychotic or depressed elderly patients who cannot tolerate any kind of drug therapy.

ECT produces results much faster than antidepressant drugs. There is temporary memory loss, but otherwise, the procedure is relatively safe. And, contrary to popular belief, it is not painful. In fact, the patient does not feel the current and experiences only minor finger or toe movements. Typically, a patient is drowsy or confused for an hour after treatment, although memory loss or difficulty in learning new material may persist for several weeks.

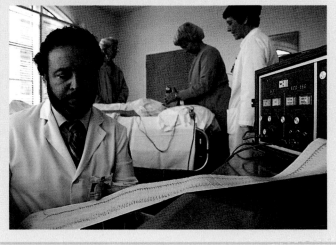

PSYCHOACTIVE DRUGS

CLASS OF DRUG	COMMON EXAMPLES	WHAT IT'S USED FOR	POTENTIAL PROBLEMS
Benzodiazepines (minor tranquilizers)	Librium (chlordiazepoxide); Valium (diazepam); Xanax (alprazolam)	Anxiety; sleep problems	Drowsiness, drug dependency, depressed respiration, especially when combined with alcohol
Neuroleptics (major tranquilizers)	Haldol (haloperidol); Largactil (chlorpromazine); Serentil (mesoridazine)	Psychotic disorders (schizophrenia, mania, severe paranoia)	Drowsiness, tics, muscle spasms, and other movement abnormalities
Barbiturates	phenobarbital, secobarbital	Sleep problems in people who cannot take benzodiazepines	Same problems as benzodiazepines, only more so; overdose can be fatal
Tricyclic antidepressants	Anafranil (clomipramine); Elavil, Levate (amitriptyline); Surmontil (trimipramine); Tofranil (imipramine)	Clinical depression	Drowsiness, dry mouth, blurred vision, difficulty urinating; overdose can be fatal
Newer antidepressants	Asendin (amoxapine); Ludiomil (maprotiline); Prozac (fluoxetine)	Clinical depression	Same as tricyclics; possible increased risk of suicide during early recovery
MAO inhibitors	Manerix (moclobemide); Nardil (phenelzine)	Clinical depression	Severe high blood pressure when taken with foods high in tyramine (e.g.,cheese, meat, red wine)
Lithium	Carbolith, Lithane, and others	Mania and manic-depression	Lithium toxicity

New or Experimental Treatments

Medical researchers constantly seek new and better treatments, especially for incurable diseases such as AIDS and cancer. Before these can be offered to humans, even on an experimental basis, they must undergo extensive testing, a process during which most are weeded out. Some turn out to be ineffective, others unsafe, and still others are not considered an improvement over existing therapies. Although the list of experimental treatments keeps changing, here are a few that look the most promising in the 1990s:

Immunotherapy

The body's immune system serves as the first line of defense against bacteria, viruses, and other potentially harmful invaders. Immunotherapy manipulates the immune system, either by suppressing or bolstering its natural function of fighting disease. Powerful drugs that suppress the immune system make organ transplantation possible by subduing the body's natural rejection of a foreign tissue.

Sometimes, the immune system goes into action against the body's healthy tissue, resulting in an autoimmune disease. Researchers are working on new immunosuppresive drugs to treat these diseases, which include chronic inflammatory disorders, such as lupus and certain other forms of arthritis.

The opposite approach, bolstering the immune system, is considered one of the most promising new medical frontiers. Several experimental cancer treatments are designed to stimulate the immune system to fight cancer in much the same way that it wards off or rejects any foreign invader. One approach is to develop vaccines against specific cancers. Another involves the use of interferon, interleukin-2, and other natural body chemicals that prompt an immune attack against tumors. Similar immunotherapy approaches are under investigation for the treatment of AIDS.

Yet another experimental cancer treatment, called transfer factor or adoptive therapy, takes a specific antibody from a healthy person and injects it into a patient who has a particular type of cancer, in the hope that it will trigger an immune system attack on the cancer cells.

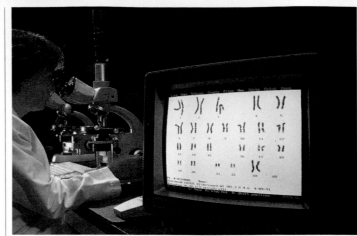

Genetic engineering represents the most hopeful prospect for overcoming hereditary diseases such as cystic fibrosis.

Genetic Engineering

Genes are the individual units of chromosomes, the body's blueprints that make it possible for cells to duplicate themselves in an orderly and consistent fashion. From time to time, genes change, or mutate. Some mutations go unnoticed, but others result in disease. Many genetic diseases, such as cystic fibrosis and muscular dystrophy, are the result of mutations that are inherited, whereas certain cancers develop when the genetic material in cells undergoes mutations during an individual's lifetime.

Environmental factors, such as radiation exposure and tobacco smoking, can prompt genetic mutations that result in disease, but many seem to occur spontaneously, without any obvious promoting factor.

Scientists are just beginning to understand how to manipulate genes to fight disease. Monoclonal antibodies are already used in experimental cancer treatments. Antibodies are the disease-fighting substances produced by the immune system. Genetic engineers can now fuse several types of antibodies—creating super antibodies—and use cloning techniques to produce large quantities of them, which are then injected into cancer patients. Some monoclonal antibodies are engineered to attack cancer cells. Others carry anticancer drugs or radioactive materials directly to the cancer cells, thereby killing them while sparing normal tissue.

Similar genetic engineering holds promise for curing or preventing hereditary diseases. For example, researchers are working on curing cystic fibrosis by getting the body to substitute a normal gene for the one that causes this deadly disease. To accomplish this, the normal gene is attached to a virus that has been rendered harmless, which then carries the gene to the lungs and other target organs. As the gene replicates itself, it replaces the defective one. In time, doctors may be able to replace disease-carrying genes with normal ones during fetal development.

Lasers

A laser, an acronym for light amplification by stimulated emission of radiation, is an extremely intense light beam that produces immense heat and power when it is focused at close range. When a laser beam is directed at any part of the body, the cells absorb its energy and convert it to heat. Almost instantly the tissue becomes charred or evaporates.

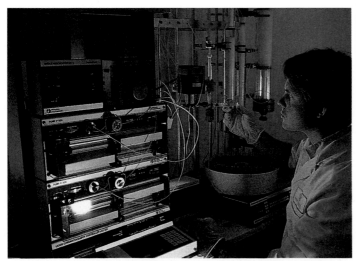

Meticulous laboratory testing is mandatory before new treatments can be offered to humans, even on a voluntary experimental basis.

Lasers have tremendous potential in surgery because they remove tissue with minimal bleeding and scarring. They are now widely used to perform delicate eye surgery, remove birthmarks and other skin blemishes, and burn off small tumors. Lasers have also proved invaluable in the treatment of female infertility due to scarring and closure of the fallopian tubes, which are the passageways between the ovary and the uterus where fertilization takes place.

Researchers believe lasers also have great potential in treating atherosclerosis, the buildup of fatty deposits, or plaque, in arteries. This type of laser surgery already is being performed experimentally to improve circulation in the legs.

Even more exciting are prospects that lasers can be used to unclog coronary arteries, the blood vessels that carry blood to the heart muscle. One approach employs laser surgery in angioplasty, a procedure in which a flexible catheter with a balloon tip is inserted into an artery and the balloon inflated to flatten any fatty deposits. Although angioplasty allows more blood to flow through the artery, it does not remove the plaque and, in time, the arteries renarrow. Researchers are working on ways to manipulate a laser device through the catheter and use its beam to vaporize the plaque. A problem is to control the light beam so it does not puncture the artery walls. But specialists at several major medical centers are now using laser angioplasty on an experimental basis.

Laser surgery employs powerful light beams that allow surgeons to perform delicate eye operations and other procedures in which bleeding and scarring must be minimized.

TESTING NEW DRUGS

In Canada, more than 50 new drugs appear on the market every year. However, before any new drug can be offered to the public, its manufacturer must prove that it is safe and effective, and to do this, its scientists have to test the drug on human beings. As it turns out, this human testing, known as clinical trials, is the most costly and time-consuming phase of drug development. Roughly 70 percent of research costs are spent on this phase.

The Testing Process

To initiate clinical tests, the manufacturer must file an Investigational New Drug Submission with the Drugs Directorate of Health Canada. This submission asks permission to distribute the new drug to responsible clinical investigators. It also contains information such as testing data up to the time of the submission and details about manufacturing methods and standards, etc.

If clinical trials prove that the new drug has potential therapeutic value that outweighs the risks associated with its use (adverse side effects, for example), the manufacturer may then file a New Drug Submission with the Drugs Directorate.

A New Drug Submission must contain the following details: the drug's proper and chemical names, its various properties, its method of manufacture. Dosage information in the submission includes: a quantitative listing of all ingredients, quality control information, therapeutic claims, clinical studies, etc. The submission can range from several pages to lengthy documents. If the New Drug Submission is satisfactory, Health Canada assigns a Drug Identification Number (DIN) and issues a Notice of Compliance, which permits the manufacturer to sell the drug.

How Human Testing Works

Health Canada itself does not conduct human testing. This is carried out by a drug manufacturer, a public or private institution (for example, a university may also sponsor some studies). But Health Canada—through its Health Protection Branch—oversees the rigorous testing process.

During the initial phase of clinical trials, an experimental drug is given to healthy volunteers for several months to make sure it is safe. During the next phase, volunteer patients take the drug for a few months to two years to determine its effectiveness and safety. For this phase, the volunteers are often divided into two or more groups, with a number receiving the new drug and others getting a placebo. In some cases, a third group may be taking an existing drug to find out if its effects are equivalent to the new one.

Only a small percentage of experimental drugs go on to the final testing phase, which typically involves several thousand patients and lasts usually for one to four years. During this period, the safety, effectiveness, and dosages are refined. Even if the drug is eventually offered to the public, it must still be monitored for adverse reactions, long-term safety, and efficacy.

How to Volunteer

Participants in clinical tests are recruited in many ways. Often a hospital, a drug company, or an agency simply advertises for participants. Doctors are sometimes enlisted to conduct clinical trials, and may use their own patients or recruit additional volunteers. Teaching hospitals also participate in clinical trials and offer both experimental drugs and treatments to selected patients.

No matter who conducts the tests, all participants must be fully informed of any risks. Participants must be given enough information about the test to make a sound decision before signing a consent form, and they must be told that they can leave the test at any time without prejudice to their rights. Volunteers are not told whether they are receiving the actual drug or a placebo, because knowing this might alter test results.

False Hopes

Desperate patients with incurable diseases often look to experimental drugs as a last resort for a cure. Some clinical studies fulfill this hope, and provide excellent medical care during the process. Others may fall short of expectations, but still succeed in advancing medical knowledge. Always be wary if you are asked to pay for an experimental drug. In such cases, ask to see evidence that Health Canada has approved the study. If the source is doubtful, check with your doctor, local hospital or the manufacturer of the drug before volunteering.

Natural Medicine

Natural, or alternative, medicine is often thought of as a phenomenon of the so-called New Age; in reality, much of it is older than human history. Every society has herbal cures and folk remedies, many of which have been incorporated into orthodox medicine. In fact, it is estimated that at least half of our modern drugs originated with natural plant sources.

In ancient times, many diseases were attributed to the supernatural—a sick person was thought to be possessed by demons or to have incurred the displeasure of some god. Thus, many treatments were aimed at exorcising demons; priests or shamans often doubled as physicians, because it was felt they could heal by restoring a god's favor.

These beliefs started to change some 3,000 years ago as Indian, Chinese, and Greek philosophers postulated that health signified a balance of internal forces, and that illness occurred when this natural harmony was upset. This idea gave rise to distinct medical systems and practices aimed at maintaining internal harmony. The alternative medicine of today is a direct outgrowth of these millenia-old medical practices, using many of the same techniques.

After the fall of the Roman Empire, a different world view—and with it, different medical practices—took hold in Europe, initiating the rift between Western and Eastern medicine. This rift widened further during the Renaissance, with the rise of scientific inquiry and the beginnings of modern scientific approaches to medicine.

In this century, North American physicians embraced scientific medicine wholeheartedly, discarding and even outlawing much of what are now considered alternative therapies. But in other parts of the world, including industrialized European nations, traditional therapies continued to coexist with mainstream medicine. Even in India, where the teaching of traditional ayurvedic medicine was banned under British rule, the practice never disappeared, and quickly reemerged when India gained its independence.

Today, growing numbers of North Americans have come to recognize that achieving and maintaining good health is a personal responsibility, affected by lifestyle. There is increasing emphasis on good nutrition, regular exercise, weight control, and smoking cessation. Many alternative therapies, which were once dismissed as mostly hokum, are now considered complimentary adjuncts to conventional medicine, important in preventing and treating many diseases.

Alternative practitioners and their patients have led the movement toward natural medicine, but several prominent U.S. physicians and medical educators, among them Dr. Bernie Segal and Dr. Andrew Weill, have helped to sway both the public and physician colleagues, often with best-selling books. Dr. Weill in particular offers a balanced approach by advocating that patients see mainstream physicians for infections and other acute illnesses, in which they can truly make a difference, and try alternative therapies for chronic problems that conventional medicine is unable to do much about.

Other well known mainstream physicians, cardiologist Dean Ornish, for instance, advocate a combination of conventional and alternative therapies plus lifestyle changes to treat even serious conditions such as heart disease. The following pages describe some of the more popular alternative therapies and their potential benefits and limitations.

Acupuncture and Other Chinese Remedies

Yin and Yang

Acupuncture is a form of healing based on the concept that all body organs are interconnected by channels, known as meridians, and that illness occurs when the vital energy, or qi (pronounced chee), flowing through these channels is partially blocked. A practitioner of acupuncture attempts to correct this imbalance by inserting thin needles along the meridians at designated points, called acupoints, and in certain cases twirling them, either manually or with an electrical device. He or she may combine the treatment with other traditional practices, such as herbal medicine, diet therapy, and massage.

The most effective acupuncturists are said to contribute their own qi during the procedure. Transmission of energy occurs when the needles are inserted and rotated.

Origins

The Chinese developed the acupuncture system over 2,000 years ago out of a principle of Taoist religious philosophy. As with all traditional Chinese medicine, it is based on the theory that good health depends upon a balance of the forces of yin and yang. These opposites, which exist in nature—as female and male, moon and sun, darkness and light—have their counterparts within the body. Illness occurs when these forces are out of sync, so the goal of this particular therapy is to restore balance.

Acupoints were designated according to their assumed clinical function in restoring the balance of yin and yang, thereby improving circulation of both qi and blood. One legend, which attempts to explain how acupoints were determined, says that during wars in ancient times, physicians observed

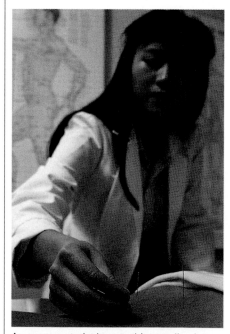
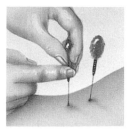
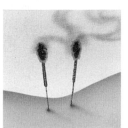

An acupuncturist inserts thin needles into specific acupoints and then twirls the needle (upper right), or applies moxa (center right), an herb that produces penetrating heat when burned (lower right).

that soldiers who had been struck by arrows in certain parts of the body were mysteriously cured of specific illnesses.

Western interest in acupuncture has developed sporadically. In the 18th century, when Christian missionaries from Europe were expelled from China, some took acupuncture techniques back home with them. In the 19th century, Chinese workers, who came to North America to help build the railroads, brought information about acupuncture, among other remedies, which ultimately caught the attention of some doctors and healers. More recently, interest in acupuncture has been sparked by two events: the opening of China to the West and the investigation of alternative methods of dealing with pain.

Practitioners

With the growing interest in acupuncture, it has been easier to find a practitioner—though not necessarily a qualified one. In Quebec, acupuncturists have been licensed since 1985. Alberta and British Columbia are considering licensing regulations. Most provinces allow physicians with acupuncture training to perform the procedure.

When it is used

While many of the claims by acupuncturists are viewed with skepticism by mainstream doctors, there is increasing recognition of their success in alleviating pain, thereby providing an alternative to painkillers, tranquilizers, and sleeping pills. The use of acupuncture for anesthesia in dentistry, childbirth, and some forms of surgery is under study by a number of Western medical practitioners. Researchers are also looking into its usefulness as a way of easing the pain and increasing the range of motion for people who suffer from rheumatoid arthritis and osteoarthritis. Other possible uses of acupuncture include the treatment of allergies, migraine headaches, circulatory disorders, and addictions to nicotine, alcohol, and other drugs.

Interest in acupuncture and other traditional Chinese remedies is increasing in North America, but their acceptance in Europe is greater. For example, acupuncture is taught in French medical schools and is covered by government health insurance in France and several other European countries.

MOXIBUSTION AND CUPPING

A major method of acupuncture therapy is moxibustion, in which the herb moxa, or mugwort, is applied directly on the skin or indirectly on the needle (see illustration, opposite page) at the acupuncture point. The use of direct moxa is prescribed in specific cases as the prime treatment.

Cupping, shown right, is another traditional Chinese procedure. Glass suction cups, or pulling cups, are placed on the acupoints and the tissues under the cup are pulled upward to stimulate increased blood flow within the cupped area. Cupping is not widely used in North America. In the past, however, immigrants from Eastern Europe used it to treat a variety of ailments.

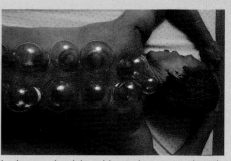

In dry cupping (above) heated cups are placed over the skin to draw tissue into them. In wet cupping, the cups are placed over small skin punctures to produce bleeding.

How it works

There is no parallel in Western medicine for the meridians and acupoints indicated on the traditional acupuncture chart. Within the frame of reference for Western science, it has not been possible to validate the claims of acupuncture as a healing system, nor is there a complete understanding of exactly how it works as an analgesic. Some researchers think its positive effects might result from the release of endorphins, the body's naturally produced analgesics, triggered by the action of the needles. Although the trigger points for pain and for acupuncture have been labeled differently and were discovered independently, recent research into pain has revealed that they represent the same phenomenon and can be explained in terms of how the nervous system functions.

What to expect

Treatment consists of the insertion of hair-thin stainless steel needles a few millimeters below the skin at specifically designated locations. The mystery is that the needles are inserted in one part of the body, yet the sensations of warmth, numbness, or tingling are experienced in another part. The traditional explanation for this phenomenon is that qi is traveling along its proper channel. Recent Western research suggests that the autonomic nervous system is responsible.

In current practice, the needles range in diameter from 10 to 13 mils (thousandths of an inch) and from one to three inches in length. It takes considerable skill and many years of practice to insert the needles perpendicular to the skin without bending them. Their insertion and removal rarely cause pain beyond the sensation of a pin prick. When the patient is relaxed, there is no discomfort at any stage of the procedure.

For treating pain, the length of time that needles are left in place, whether they are twirled manually or hooked up to an electrical rotating device, and whether the acupuncture is combined with heat, depends on the nature of the pain or the desired effect. For example, 5 minutes is said to be sufficient for tooth extraction, while 20 to 30 minutes may be needed for a tonsillectomy, with continuous stimulation by the needles throughout the entire surgical procedure. In the last instance, the analgesic effect lasts about 24 hours.

Most treatments for pain relief take 5 to 15 minutes. Since the effect is presumed to be cumulative, a course of six treatments is usually recommended. Some patients, whose pain has not been alleviated immediately after treatment, report its disappearance days or even weeks later.

Precautions

▶ Anyone contemplating acupuncture should be medically assessed before beginning treatment.

▶ Unless your acupuncturist is a licensed M.D. or D.O., or has been recommended by your primary-care doctor, check credentials and training.

▶ Acupuncturists generally sterilize their needles with wet heat (autoclave). Because AIDS, hepatitis B, and other deadly diseases can be transmitted by contaminated needles, however, reuse of needles—even after autoclaving—should be avoided. Disposable needles are available at very low cost.

Alexander Technique

The Alexander technique is a training process in which a person learns to identify and change faulty posture and movements. The goal is to free the body of muscular tensions that cause stress and fatigue by eliminating common postural problems resulting from such habits as slouching, holding the head in an awkward position when talking on the telephone, or carrying a heavy bag on one shoulder.

A number of poor posture patterns are the result of well-intentioned reminders by parents or teachers to stand or sit up straight. Many people respond by holding their spinal muscles in a constant state of tension instead of aiming for a relaxed balance of head, neck, and torso. Tight or restrictive clothing and high heeled shoes are other common culprits that contribute to incorrect posture and muscle tension.

Origins

The technique was developed in the late 19th century by an Australian actor, F. Mathias Alexander, during a period in his career when he was losing his voice. While examining his movements in a triple mirror, he realized that the tense and artificial postures he habitually assumed with his head, neck, and torso during performances were affecting his vocal chords. By changing his self-defeating habits, he was able to "liberate" his voice.

Encouraged by his success, he began to teach others some of his methods and in 1908, he published one of his earliest pamphlets: "Re-education of the Kinesthetic System (Sensory Appreciation of Muscular Movement) Concerned with the

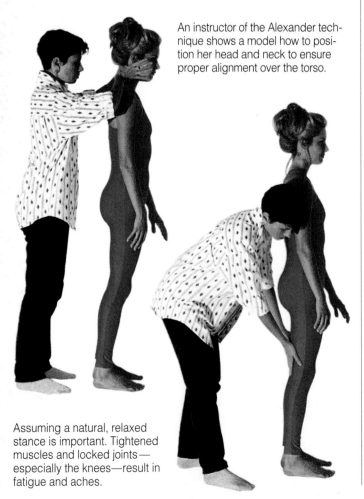

An instructor of the Alexander technique shows a model how to position her head and neck to ensure proper alignment over the torso.

Assuming a natural, relaxed stance is important. Tightened muscles and locked joints — especially the knees—result in fatigue and aches.

Precautions
► Ascertain that a teacher of the Alexander technique has the proper training and certification .
► Find out about payment arrangements before committing yourself to a series of lessons.

Development of Robust Physical Well-Being." In the decades that followed, he attracted many distinguished followers, among them philosopher John Dewey, authors George Bernard Shaw and Aldous Huxley, as well as a number of physicians and scientists. By the time he died in 1955, his technique was being taught worldwide.

Practitioners

Instructors are trained and certified at centers affiliated with the North American Society of Teachers of the Alexander Technique. They may give private lessons and also conduct group classes and workshops.

Some doctors and physical therapists use the method, and many hospitals, rehabilitation centers, and pain clinics now offer instruction to their clients. So do performing arts institutions, including the Juilliard School in New York and the London Academy of Music and Dramatic Arts.

When it is used

The technique is most frequently recommended as a way of dealing with back and neck pain. It is also used to counteract some of the effects of scoliosis (curvature of the spine) and arthritis, to improve respiratory function, and as an adjunct to breathing exercises for asthma patients.

Some performing artists claim that it has helped them to overcome stage fright; many athletes have found that it not only enhances their skills but also helps reduce the likelihood of sports injuries. A growing number of people who work at computers are investigating the Alexander technique as a way of avoiding stress injuries from repetitive movements, which have become a disabling occupational hazard.

How it works

The Alexander technique is based on the assumption that the body can move freely and naturally only when the head, neck, and torso are properly aligned. This requires awareness of faulty muscular movements and correction of them.

What to expect

Teaching sessions usually last from 30 to 45 minutes. Their number is determined by the severity of the problem and how quickly the person learns to correct it. Typically, 10 to 15 classes are sufficient to address most problems.

During one of the first lessons, the student may be told to lie on a padded table while the instructor discusses ways in which the body parts relate to each other. The goal is to help the person achieve a natural rest position that can be practiced at home. Then the student's body is observed as she goes about ordinary tasks—rising from a chair, speaking on the telephone, carrying a pile of books, lifting a heavy carton from the floor. During each of these exercises, the instructor uses a hands-on approach to explore the neck and shoulders of the student for signs of muscle tension. At the same time, the instructor points out faulty movements so that they can be corrected. Critical assessment of posture and movement is often made in front of a mirror so that the client can see the difference between bad habits and better ones.

Aromatherapy

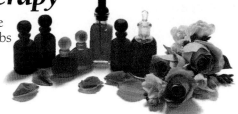

Aromatherapy is the use of oils from herbs and other aromatic plants to achieve relaxation or relief from a disorder. Depending upon the plant, the aromatic, or essential, oil is extracted from the leaves, flowers, roots, seeds, fruit, bark, or resin and then diluted with water or an unscented oil such as jojoba. These solutions may be massaged into skin, inhaled from steam, added to bath water, or used in a compress.

Origins

Aromatic plants, usually applied externally, have been used in many folk remedies since ancient times. Familiar examples include vaporized eucalyptus oil to ease nasal congestion and juniper liniment for the relief of muscle aches.

Modern aromatherapy was born in the 1920s, when a French chemist, Dr. René-Maurice Gattefossé, burned his hand while working in a perfume laboratory. He plunged the injured hand into a container of lavender oil and was amazed by its speedy healing with minimal scarring. He then began to research the healing properties of other aromatic oils.

Practitioners

Aromatherapy is used by trained therapists who often practice other alternative therapies such as massage. Some of the methods can be self-taught and used at home.

When it is used

Practitioners treat a range of medical and emotional problems, including headaches, premenstrual tension, muscle pain, skin disorders, fatigue, insomnia, and stress.

Precautions

▶ Avoid ingesting aromatic oils used for aromatherapy. Many, such as camphor and yellow jasmine, are highly toxic. Make sure that the oils are stored in a safe place out of children's reach.
▶ Many aromatic oils are highly irritating, especially when used in concentrated amounts or on the delicate membranes of the vagina, rectum, or nasal cavities. Follow directions for diluting the oils, and then test the diluted solution on a small patch of skin on the forearm or thigh. Avoid further use if the oil produces redness, itching, or swelling.

How it works

There are two basic mechanisms involved—the sense of smell and the absorptive quality of skin. Practitioners contend that inhalation of a certain scent prompts the brain to release neurochemicals that counter stress and fatigue. They also believe that some oils exert a medicinal effect when absorbed by the skin. Medical benefits of aromatherapy have not been proven, however, and doctors generally discount any therapeutic benefits other than a placebo effect and relaxation.

What to expect

Aromatherapists combine massage and the use of aromatic oils. A session varies according to the problem being treated. The entire body is massaged to relieve stress and general achiness. A facial massage is used to treat headaches and sinus congestion, whereas the back may be massaged to alleviate backache or menstrual cramps.

In addition to massage, an aromatherapist may recommend soaking in a tub of warm water containing a few drops of one or more aromatic oils. Depending upon the oils used, this may induce drowsiness or provide an invigorating lift.

EXAMPLES OF AROMATIC OILS

OIL	SOURCE	WHAT IT'S USED FOR
Chamomile	Dried flowers	Mild, sweet, grain-like aroma. Used in vaporizers, baths, compresses, facial masks, or massages for its soothing effects; also said to speed healing of minor burns, alleviate eczema, and ease muscle pain.
Clary sage	Flowering tops	Strong, pungent aroma. Inhaled or used in vaporizers, baths, compresses, or massages to alleviate anxiety, stress, skin inflammation, and respiratory congestion.
Eucalyptus	Leaves	Strong, invigorating, camphor-like aroma. Used in vaporizers, compresses, baths, and massages to treat nasal and respiratory congestion, alleviate muscle pain, and counter fatigue; applied to the skin as an insect repellant.
Geranium	Leaves	Sharp, spicy fragrance. Used in vaporizers, baths, massages, and (less commonly) mouthwashes and gargles; considered a basic oil to treat stress, acne, eczema, and minor wounds.
Jasmine	Flowers	Subtle floral aroma. Used in facial massages and baths for its relaxing properties.
Juniper berry	Ripe berries	Sharp, peppery fragrance. Used in vaporizers, baths, compresses, and massages for its calming effect; aromatherapists also use it to treat muscle aches and eczema.
Lavender	Flowering tops	Strong, sweet floral fragrance. Used in vaporizers, baths, compresses, and massages to treat stress and skin wounds; said to have antiseptic and anti-inflammatory properties.
Peppermint	Leaves	Fresh, invigorating aroma. Inhaled or used in baths, gargles, and mouthwashes for digestive upsets, sore throat, mouth ulcers, and itchy skin; also used as an insect repellant.
Pine	Resin	Invigorating wood scent. Used in vaporizers, baths, and massages to alleviate muscle aches and treat nasal and chest congestion.
Rose	Flowers	Delicate, persistent floral fragrance. Used in baths and massages for its relaxing qualities. Aromatherapists also use it to treat menstrual problems and other female reproductive disorders.

Art Therapy

Art therapy is the use of visual arts materials to identify and treat emotional trauma and mental disorders. By creating images in drawings, paintings, sculptures, and photographs, patients provide information about suppressed feelings and buried memories that they cannot express with words.

This approach is also an important aspect of rehabilitation programs for people who are recovering from a stroke or an injury affecting hand function. It can help disabled people to improve their self-image and depressed or elderly patients to expand their range of expression.

Origins

The term art therapy was first used in the 1940s to describe the work of U.S. psychiatrists and psychologists who were finding that artistic expression provided important insight into the feelings of disturbed children. Independent practitioners eventually established the American Art Therapy

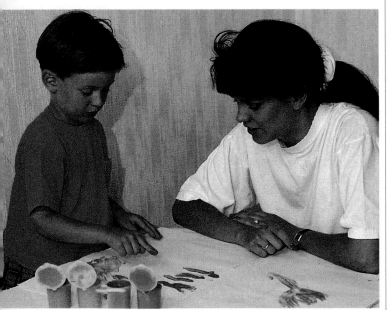

An art therapist encourages a young patient to use finger painting to express feelings that are difficult to put into words.

Association, which issued guidelines for the first formal training program in the late 1960s.

In 1967, the late Martin Fischer established the Toronto Art Therapy Institute. A decade later, the institute became the headquarters for the nationwide Canadian Art Therapy Association, which initiated its training program at that time. By the early 1990s, there were about 500 Canadian art therapists, based mainly in Ontario, British Columbia, and Quebec.

An important recent development in the field of art therapy has been the formation of Medart International, an organization that investigates and promotes the relationship between established medicine and the visual and performing arts.

Practitioners

In Canada, most art therapists enter their field from university programs in art of psychology. Concordia University in Montreal is the only university in Canada offering a master's degree in art therapy. The Canadian Art Therapy Association registers, but does not license, its therapists.

Precautions
► All art materials used in a therapeutic setting, especially by children, should be nontoxic.
► People with allergies should be especially careful about the contents of paints and solvents.

When it is used

Art therapy is used with patients who cannot or will not employ words to achieve the personal insight that is a cornerstone of traditional psychotherapy. By surmounting language barriers, this therapy can be especially effective with disturbed children and patients who speak a different language from the therapist. It is also helpful in rehabilitating hand/motor skills following a stroke or injury and assessing the progress of a patient by comparing an early attempt at a self-portrait with a similar attempt after physical therapy.

How it works

By providing a patient with a nonverbal means of expressing repressed thoughts and feelings, art therapy can help ease guilt and anger. Sexually abused children often render images whose meaning can eventually be discussed. Through drawings and paintings, a schizophrenic patient may offer the therapist a view into a disordered mind, thus providing some clues for how treatment might proceed.

Art therapy can also enable mentally ill deaf adults to describe early conflicts with family members and to alleviate symptoms of aggression, hostility, and depression. Physically handicapped children, neglected elderly persons, alcoholics, and prison inmates all can be helped to build self-esteem through sculpture, painting, or photography, especially when they see their work exhibited for other people's appreciation.

What to expect

Through supportive discussions with an art therapist, patients become aware of the messages conveyed in their drawings, paintings, or sculptures. When previously unacknowledged frustration, rage, or confusion has been brought to light, the patient can be helped to take positive steps for dealing with it. Practiced in a family setting, art therapy can also resolve interpersonal problems.

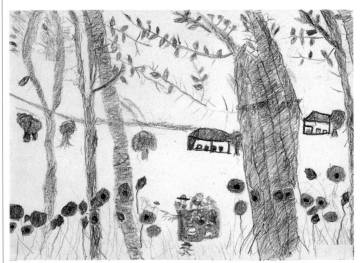

Art therapy can help a stroke patient, such as the creator of this picture, with visual organization, memory, and concentration.

Ayurveda

This ancient healing system from India stresses the mind/body relationship in the maintenance of good health. As in other Asian medical practices, a balance of vital energy, in this case, prana, is considered the key. The system is based on balancing three basic life forces, or doshas—vata, responsible for all movement in the body; pitta, which controls digestion and energy production; and kapha, responsible for the body's structure and stability. Illness occurs when any of the doshas is out of sync; individuals must know their dominant dosha and follow a diet and lifestyle that keeps it balanced with the others.

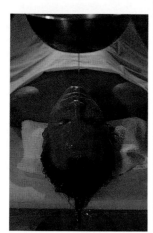

During an ayurvedic session, a warm aromatic oil is poured over the skin, which is then massaged.

Origins
Ayurveda, meaning the "science of life and longevity" in Sanskrit, is believed to be about 5,000 years old, predating all other medical systems. The two classic Ayurveda textbooks are more than 2,000 years old. *Charaka Samhita,* named for the person who was the ayurvedic counterpart of Hippocrates, outlines the principles of health maintenance and treatment of disease, and *Sushruta Samhita* describes elaborate surgical procedures, including reconstructive plastic surgery, gallbladder removal, and other operations that most people consider modern.

Ayurvedic medicine spread with the Hindu culture to Indonesia, Tibet, and eventually to the West, where some of its principles were picked up by the ancient Greek physicians. As Buddhism developed, this healing system was carried to China and other Asian countries.

During the 1800s, the British banned all ayurvedic schools in India, replacing them with Western medical schools. For the next century, ayurvedic medicine was relegated to folk practices in rural areas. When India regained its independence in 1947, ayurvedic schools were again legalized. Today, there are 100 ayurvedic schools in India, equal in number to the Western ones, and many Indian physicians incorporate both styles of medicine into their practices.

In recent years, Ayurveda has spread to North America. There are major clinics in the United States, and some consultation centers exist in Toronto, Montreal, and Ottawa.

Practitioners
In India, Ayurveda practitioners must undergo five to six years of training in a traditional ayurvedic medical school before they can treat patients. In the United States, this training is abbreviated into a short course of several months at an ayurvedic institute. Whichever training they have received, ayurvedic physicians are not licensed to practice medicine here, unless they are trained also in another discipline, such as traditional medicine, osteopathy, or chiropractic.

When it is used
Unlike Western medicine, which comes into play when illness strikes, Ayurveda is incorporated into a person's lifestyle. It governs all aspects of life, such as diet, exercise, and sexual practices. An ayurvedic practitioner is consulted only to identify and correct an imbalance among the three life forces. At ayurvedic clinics in the United States, patients are usually treated by both a Western and an ayurvedic physician.

How it works
Ayurvedic philosophy holds that each person is born with a particular ratio of doshas, with one dominating. This dominant dosha determines personality type and also influences one's susceptibility to certain illnesses. For example, pitta people tend to have fiery dispositions and are prone to developing high blood pressure and digestive disorders, so a pitta-related disease may be treated with a bland diet and numerous herbal remedies. Because the mind is seen as an integral force in maintaining health and overcoming illness, meditation or yoga may also be employed.

What to expect
An ayurvedic doctor begins by assessing the patient's dosha pattern. Pulses play a critical role in this assessment—a practitioner feels pulses throughout the body, looking for dosha imbalances as reflected in the nature of a pulse. Seven types of body tissue—plasma, red blood cells, muscle, fat, bone, nerve, and reproductive tissue—are also examined.

Ayurvedic physicians do not focus on a specific disease or an organ system, but instead treat the entire body and mind. Purification to rid the body of toxins is an important part of treatment; methods may include sweat baths, enemas, nasal washes, bloodletting, and oil massages. The practitioner will also recommend a specific diet, meditation or yoga routine, and herbal remedies.

Precautions
▶ Before agreeing to ayurvedic treatments, ask about costs and cancellation policies. Some clincis ask for advance payment and require two week's notice of cancellation to qualify for a refund.

THE SPA EXPERIENCE
For centuries, health enthusiasts have journeyed to special locales such as the Belgian town of Spa to partake of fresh air, healing waters, and a variety of traditional and nontraditional medical treatments. Today, spas remain an integral part of health care in many European countries, where national health plans often pay for a sojourn in a preventive or therapeutic medical facility that may look more like a luxury resort than a clinic.

Spas have gained popularity in North America as well, although insurance companies are unlikely to pay for their services. Still, those who can afford the fees (which range from $1,000 to $4,000 per week) stand to benefit from a spa visit. Most spas in North America provide low-fat meals, exercise and meditation classes, and massage and other body therapies. Popular spas, some relaxed and indulgent and others run with the no-nonsense rigor of an army camp, are typically located in scenic areas; the settings themselves often have a salutary effect.

A growing number of spas address specific medical problems, such as hypertension, obesity, and heart disease. Still others approach health promotion from the perspective of a particular discipline. In general, though, some of the best spas draw on a variety of disciplines, including traditional Western medicine. As such, they focus less on treating illness than on giving visitors the feeling of healthful living—an experience that they can, ideally, carry forward after returning home.

Biofeedback Training

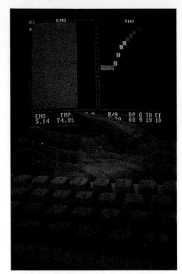

Electronic sensors and signals are utilized to teach a person how to control bodily functions, such as blood flow, that normally are automatic or involuntary.

Biofeedback training allows a person to gain a measure of control over bodily functions that are usually automatic, or involuntary—for example, heartbeat, blood pressure, skin temperature, blood flow to the hands and feet, even brain-wave patterns. Some doctors believe that the results are similar to those of self-hypnosis.

Electronic monitors used to measure these responses produce visible or audible signals. During the training, a person learns how to alter the electronic signals and, in the process, change an involuntary bodily response.

Origins

In the early years of radio, the term "feedback" was created to describe the design principle that enabled electronic systems to self-correct through an information loop. Biofeedback training applies this principle to the correction, or self-regulation, of one's own biological systems.

Experiments in applying biofeedback principles to the body were conducted as part of dream-sleep studies in the late 1950s. The subjects were trained to produce alpha brain-wave patterns, which indicate a mental state of relaxed alertness, on an electroencephalograph screen.

Eventually, scientists at the Menninger Foundation in Topeka, Kansas, were able to teach patients how to alleviate their migraine headaches by redirecting some of the blood flow from constricted blood vessels in the scalp to their hands. To do this, patients were instructed to concentrate on raising their hand temperature by visualizing holding something warm, such as a cup of hot coffee. Since then, biofeedback training has been used to treat numerous ailments.

Practitioners

The training may be done by a physician, psychologist, physical therapist, or laboratory technician, often in a rehabilitation center or a pain clinic.

When it is used

Common uses are to control pain, relieve asthma attacks, rehabilitate muscles damaged by stroke or accident, and treat insomnia, migraine headaches, and other stress-related conditions. Biofeedback training is often combined with visualization and breathing exercises. Researchers in a heart attack prevention program at Duke University in Durham, North Carolina, have used the training to modify Type A personality traits, especially persistent feelings of anger and hostility, which are thought to increase the risk of heart attack.

In some cases, biofeedback can help eliminate the need for medications such as tranquilizers or prescription painkillers. In other instances, such as the control of high blood pressure, it may be combined with medication.

How it works

The goal of biofeedback training is to teach individuals how to become active participants in their own treatment, even though they may be unaware of actually controlling a bodily function. A classic example of how the process works is the experiment, conducted in 1970 at Harvard Medical School, in which male subjects were taught to modify their blood pressure. Success in decreasing their blood pressure and maintaining it at a lower level was indicated by a flashing light; after 20 such flashes, the reward was a glimpse of a nude pinup. Most of the subjects indicated that they had no awareness of actually controlling the flashing lights, nor were they conscious of what response was being measured. However, they were aware of the nude picture.

Some researchers believe that biofeedback contributes to improved physical and mental health because it fosters a feeling of power over bodily functions that were assumed to be beyond one's conscious control. Thus, even if a cure is not achieved, biofeedback training adds an important sense of well-being that may increase the efficacy of medical therapy.

What to expect

Electronic monitors are used to measure specific physical responses; the types of monitors most commonly employed during biofeedback training are:
▶ Electromyograph (EMG), which monitors muscular tension and electrical activity in the muscles.
▶ Electroencephalograph (EEG), which records brain waves.
▶ Skin temperature monitor, which senses minute changes that indicate shifts in blood flow.

The type of disorder over which the patient seeks control determines the kind of monitor used. For example, if a person wants to reduce muscle tension that is causing severe neck pain, EMG electrodes are placed on the muscles in question. These electrodes convert electrical activity of the muscles into a visual image on a screen or into audio signals heard through earphones. The therapist then teaches the patient how to change the signals to reduce the muscle tension. Similarly, by learning to control changes recorded by the EEG, a person can help manage stress, pain, insomnia, and in some cases, epileptic seizures.

Temperature monitors, which sense even slight fluctuations in skin temperature due to changes in blood flow, help patients learn to abort a migraine headache during the early warning stage. They also help people who suffer from circulatory disorders reduce the discomfort of cold hands and feet.

At first, simply seeing the image or hearing the signal is all that is needed to relax muscles or alter blood flow. Eventually, a patient is able to achieve desired results without the presence of a monitor. With practice, people can become increasingly skilled at controlling these involuntary processes.

Precautions
▶ Be wary of mail-order or other sources of biofeedback equipment to use at home because such devices vary in quality. Also, a trained therapist can teach you the most effective techniques, something you do not get with a do-it-yourself approach.
▶ Check with your doctor before undergoing biofeedback training, especially if you have a chronic disorder such as diabetes or high blood pressure. Biofeedback training can alter the need for some medications, and dosages may need to be adjusted.

Chiropractic

Chiropractic is a system of treatment based on the belief that the foundation of good health is the unhampered flow of nerve impulses that originate in the brain and spinal cord and then travel to all parts of the body. Therapy begins with analyzing the patient's spinal column for abnormal alignments of the vertebrae. When such misalignments, called subluxations, are located, they are corrected by manipulation to restore the normal flow of nerve impulses. Many chiropractors also make recommendations about nutrition and exercise, but they do not prescribe drugs or do surgery.

Origins

Energetic hands-on therapy was widely practiced by ancient healers, and manipulation of the backbone is still common in a number of cultures. In an independent movement in the United States, a systematic method of spinal manipulation was developed at the end of the 19th century by a healer in Iowa named Daniel David Palmer. In 1895, he gained local fame by curing a janitor's deafness when he manipulated a displaced vertebra. Following this success, Palmer devoted himself to refining his method of spinal treatments.

One of Palmer's early patients described his technique as "chiropractic," Greek for "accomplished by hand." The word caught on and The Palmer Infirmary and Chiropractic Institute was established in Davenport, Iowa, as a teaching and treatment center. In 1913, the year that Palmer died, Kansas became the first American state to license chiropractic healers.

It is only in recent years that this alternative therapy has overcome charges of quackery by the medical establishment. While it is not unusual for physicians such as orthopedists and rehabilitation specialists to refer patients to a chiropractor, there are still many mainstream doctors who feel that this treatment has the potential for doing more harm than good.

Even so, chiropractic seems to be attracting more patients than ever, due to an increase in sports injuries and the recent growth in musculoskeletal problems resulting from working at computers. In Canada, visits to chiropractors are covered by some provincial health plans and many private health insurance plans.

Practitioners

Chiropractors are now licensed in all Canadian provinces, and there are two training centers, one in Toronto and another in Trois-Rivières. Studies stress the biomedical sciences and provide special training in manipulation techniques. At the succesful completion of training, the graduate receives a doctor of chiropractic, or D.C., degree. Of the approximately 4,000 chiropractors in Canada, about 3,500 belong to the Canadian Chiropractic Association, the national organization. Most provinces also have their own chiropractic associations.

Years ago, many chiropractors believed spinal manipulation to be the preferred treatment for virtually every ailment. In recent decades, most have come to recognize the limitations of their therapy; they see their work as yet another way to deal with health problems. The majority of chiropractors consider themselves "mixers," who provide a holistic service that includes counseling about nutrition, exercise, and other lifestyle issues in addition to manipulations. A minority are "straights," who follow a strict philosophy of musculoskeletal adjustments.

When it is used

Most people consult a chiropractor because of pain that appears to originate in the musculoskeletal system, usually the neck and/or back. For some patients, the pain has come on suddenly, resulting from an injury on the job, in an automobile accident, or while participating in a sport. For others, the pain may be chronic, perhaps the cumulative effect of years of poor posture, a sedentary lifestyle, and increasing weight. Still others may be suffering from job-related muscle and skeletal problems, such as repetitive stress injuries. Individuals with vague, persistent symptoms such as fatigue and headaches also consult chiropractors for both spinal manipulation and counseling on nutrition and exercise.

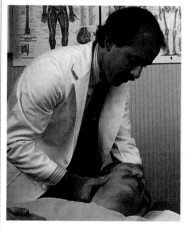

Before attempting adjustments or realignment of vertebrae, a chiropractor rotates the head and neck, feeling for tight muscles and tender points. One manipulative technique involves a rapid motion to increase joint mobility and reduce muscle spasms and pain.

Chiropractic manipulations are said to affect the 31 pairs of nerves that arise from the spinal cord and carry messages between the brain and the rest of the body.

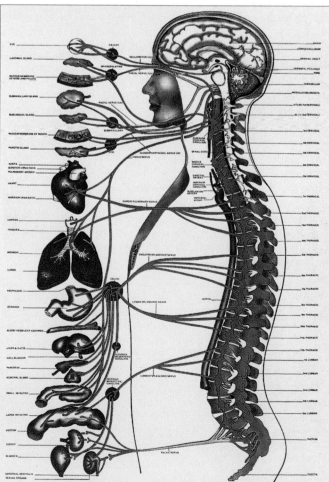

CHIROPRACTIC (CONTINUED)

How it works

The spinal cord gives rise to 31 pairs of spinal nerves, which carry messages to and from the brain and to all parts of the body. These spinal nerves pass through openings in the vertebrae, and when the progress of a nerve is impeded, it is said to be "pinched." The problem may be the result of an injury, a muscle spasm, a slipped (ruptured) vertebral disk, spinal arthritis, or some other structural abnormality.

With X-rays plus a hands-on exploration of the spine, the chiropractor tries to locate the vertebrae that need realignment. The chiropractic method is most successful in cases in which it is possible to restore normal joint movement by improving anatomical relationships. The intimate hands-on approach may also have a positive effect on healing.

Many practitioners believe that chiropractic can be most effective in treating acute pain of recent onset, before it has reached a chronic stage. Some researchers theorize that when pain is allowed to become chronic, the body loses its ability to produce endorphins, body chemicals that act as natural painkillers. This theory is based on the notion that long-term overstimulation of nerves, which occurs in chronic pain, prevents them from triggering production of painkilling chemicals.

What to expect

A visit to a chiropractor involves many of the same steps as a visit to a traditional physician. The evaluation begins with taking the patient's medical history, including questions about symptoms, past illnesses and injuries, and stresses from one's job or other situations. This is followed by a physical examination that includes blood pressure measurement, orthopedic and postural testing, a study of posture and spinal motion, and a series of X-rays. Most of these procedures may take up the entire first visit. Before the second visit, the practitioner has evaluated all this information and is ready to start treatment.

To begin, the patient lies down on a specially designed table. Muscles may be energetically massaged before manipulative techniques are used for spinal adjustment, which often produces a popping sound similar to that of cracking your knuckles. Because certain manipulative techniques involve quick, rapid motion, some transient discomfort may be experienced, especially in acute cases.

Sometimes electrical devices are employed that produce muscle fatigue to alleviate muscle spasms. Moist heat may also be applied, especially if there are muscle spasms. When it's appropriate, a supportive collar, brace, or sling may be recommended for use between treatments. Most sessions last no longer than 45 minutes, and the number of sessions depends on the nature of the problem.

Precautions
▶ Be wary of chiropractors who describe themselves as holistic healers and make extravagant claims for their cures.
▶ Do not substitute chiropractic for traditional medical treatment of heart disease, cancer, diabetes, and other organic disorders.
▶ Before undergoing X-rays in a chiropractor's office, make sure the equipment is up-to-date to minimize radiation exposure.
▶ Chiropractic treatments are generally safe for everyone, but there are exceptions. Patients who have osteoporosis and other disorders characterized by weak or brittle bones should avoid it.

The Special Niche of Osteopathy

Osteopathy is often confused with chiropractic because of its focus on manipulation. Its practitioners are fully qualified doctors, whose range covers all aspects of medicine. In the United States, osteopathy is the most widely accepted form of alternative health care, but in Canada its status is much less important.

Origins

The system was developed in the late 1800s by Andrew Taylor Still, a country doctor, to overcome what he perceived as shortcomings of orthodox medicine at that time. In 1892, he founded the American School of Osteopathy in Kirksville, Missouri, and many of his principles are still followed.

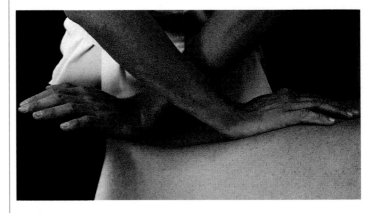

Practitioners

In Canada, osteopaths are licensed in all provinces except Manitoba, New Brunswick, Newfoundland, and Prince Edward Island. But licensing does not necessarily mean that osteopaths have the same privileges as M.D.s. Moreover, there are only a few provinces where osteopathic treatment is covered by any form of insurance.

How it works

Osteopathy is based on the premise that all organ systems form an interrelated whole, and that good health reflects a harmonic balance among organs, as well as harmony of mind and body. Any dysfunction of one part is thought to affect the entire organism adversely. Thus, treatment is directed to finding and correcting the underlying cause of the disorder.

What to expect

In making a diagnosis and formulating a treatment plan, an osteopath concentrates on the neuro-musculoskeletal system. After taking a medical history, he or she spends considerable time feeling and palpating the patient's body, looking for inflammation, tenderness, and muscle tightness or spasms. X-rays and tests may be ordered. Treatment often includes manipulation and massage, especially if there is pain.

Osteopaths can prescribe drugs and perform surgery, but they rely on these modalities less often than other doctors do. Even when prescribing drugs, osteopaths will also perform manipulations to increase the effectiveness of the medication. They will also instruct patients on good posture and exercise.

Dance Therapy

Dance therapy, also called dance/movement therapy, employs movement instead of spoken communication to treat the mentally ill. It is also used to enrich the lives of sightless and deaf individuals, especially children, and can be an important aspect of rehabilitation following a stroke or an injury that hinders motion and coordination.

Origins

While dance and movement have long been used for expression, recreation, and religious rituals, the foundation of the present therapy was laid shortly after World War I, when the pioneers in modern dance began to create choreography that expressed inner emotions. At about the same time, new approaches to the treatment of mental illness were developing and therapists increasingly recognized the importance of using body movement as an outlet for emotions that could not be expressed with words.

An early practitioner of dance therapy was Marian Chace, a dance teacher. Having observed that physical movement helped emotionally disturbed children, she began to emphasize their needs for expression rather than their mastery of technique. In the 1940s, a psychiatrist who was impressed with Chace's results invited her to work with mentally ill patients at St. Elizabeth's Hospital in Washington, D.C. In the years that followed, she received widespread recognition for her accomplishments. She had demonstrated that through dance and movement, patients previously considered hopelessly regressed and withdrawn were able to engage in group activities and take the first steps toward expressing their feelings, even if they were unable to do so verbally.

Other dance therapists appeared in the United States with a variety of techniques. In 1966, the American Dance Therapy Association was established to set standards for the profession and now has about 1,000 members. In Canada, there is no equivalent association for dance therapy.

Practitioners

In the United States, dance therapists must undergo training in a graduate level program approved by the American Dance Therapy Association. Those who complete a program can apply for entry level certification as Dance Therapist Registered (DTR), which indicates that the individual has a master's degree and is qualified to work with a team or under supervision in a professional setting. After two years of clinical practice, the therapist can apply for advanced certification with the association's Academy of Dance Therapists Registered (ADTR). This designation confirms that the holder is qualified to teach, provide supervision, and engage in private practice.

When it is used

Dance/movement therapists work with individuals who have social, emotional, cognitive, and/or physical problems. They practice in psychiatric hospitals, community day care and mental health centers, correctional facilities, rehabilitation

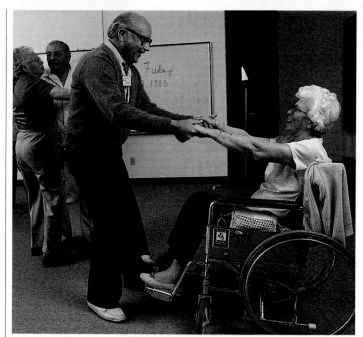

Even a patient confined to a wheelchair can benefit from the social interaction and movement of dance therapy. For others, it can be an important aspect of physical and emotional rehabilitation.

centers, clinics, nursing homes, and geriatric centers. Their work in these last two places is especially important among patients with Alzheimer's disease and others who may be incapable of ordinary social interaction. Some sports coaches also use dance therapy to improve their athletes' agility.

How it works

Participants are encouraged to overcome muscular tensions and to become aware of the way in which their feelings can affect their muscles. With the development of this awareness, they become increasingly capable of the wordless expression of inner feelings in the form of movement, usually accompanied by music. As the therapy progresses, the movements can later be interpreted and discussed.

What to expect

Patients are guided to use their bodies in movements that the therapist is trained to interpret. Through rhythmic body language, for example, an autistic child may achieve a sense of physical order that can have a healing effect on the disordered mind and feelings.

Dance therapy employed to help children with movement disorders, such as cerebral palsy, has multiple goals: to help them gain strength, improve coordination, and experience enjoyable movement free from fear of failure. The same goals apply to an older stroke patient or accident victim as well.

Individuals who are withdrawn can achieve a feeling of connectedness through holding hands in a group and facing other participants. Dance and movement can also have a positive role in the emotional and physical recovery of patients who have survived serious automobile accidents, severe burn injuries, or other mishaps that require lengthy rehabilitation and that could leave a permanent disability.

As therapy progresses, patients may be given an assignment to work on by themselves between sessions, or they may be instructed to prepare a dance improvisation for the therapist and the group to interpret.

Precautions

▶ If you are seeking a qualified dance/movement therapist for personal consultation, you can contact the American Dance Therapy Association, 200 Century Plaza, Columbia, Maryland 21044.

Herbal Medicine

Herbal medicine is the use of plants—their leaves, stems, bark, flowers, fruits, and seeds—to prevent or cure disease.

Origins

The practice probably originated in prehistoric times when humans discovered, through trial and error, that certain plants had healing powers. During the ancient civilizations of China, Egypt, Persia, and Greece, herbal remedies were codified and, eventually, compiled into books.

With the development of chemistry and the refinement of laboratory methods, herbal medicine gave way to the modern pharmaceutical industry where many drugs are created in test tubes. Still, plant-based ingredients are found in almost half of all prescription and over-the counter medications used in conventional medicine, including aspirin, digitalis, and atropine, as well as several anticancer medications.

Herbal medicine in China has for centuries been a well-organized system of knowledge based on observations, experiments, and clinical trials, and the effectiveness of a significant number of these remedies has been verified by modern science. Elsewhere, the latest effort in plant codification has been undertaken by a consortium of medical researchers, pharmaceutical companies, and herbalists who are investigating the flora of the rain forests in the hope of discovering new plant sources that might yield cures for serious diseases.

Practitioners

Herbal medicine is the specialty of people who call themselves herbalists. It is also part of homeopathy, naturopathy, and aromatherapy, as well as the mainstay of self-styled holistic healers, some with acceptable credentials, many without. Chinese herbal medicine is being popularized in the West by acupuncturists and other practitioners of Eastern medicine.

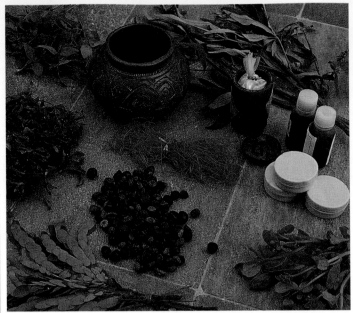

Herbs for medicines are usually dried to preserve their oils and other healing ingredients, then brewed into teas or decoctions (page 45).

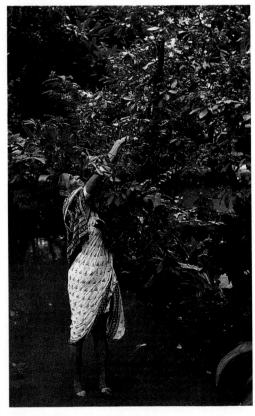

Gathering native herbs is an increasingly important pursuit in many tropical countries where rainforests are rapidly disappearing. Some major pharmaceutical companies are studying these herbs in search of ever more effective drugs.

Many salespeople in health food stores also consider themselves qualified to recommend the use of herbal extracts. Finally, many home remedies rely upon herbal preparations.

When it is used

For practitioners of herbal medicine, especially Chinese herbalists, there is a plant remedy for almost every disorder. In general, herbs are effective for treating minor ailments such as digestive problems, flu, cough, headache, and rash.

How it works

Herbal medicines that bring about a desired result are found in laboratory analyses to contain substances that trigger specific biochemical responses. For example, the inner bark of a certain type of willow tree chewed by some native peoples in North America to alleviate headaches contains salicylic acid, the active ingredient of aspirin. Some herbalists still recommend white willow to treat pain, contending that it is less likely to produce the adverse side effects of aspirin.

Health Canada recognizes herbal remedies, but it does not endorse them. An herbal remedy can be sold as an over-the-counter drug, provided it has an approved non-prescription claim and a Drug Identification Number (DIN). In granting

POISONOUS HERBS

Many herbs are highly toxic, even in small doses. Be cautious of homemade remedies, and if you gather wild herbs, be sure you know what you are picking. The following herbs can be fatal:

Aconite	Lobelia
American and black hellebore	Mayapple (European mandrake)
Arnica	
Autumn crocus	Pokeweed
Belladonna (deadly nightshade)	Rue
Bloodroot	Sassafras
Colts foot	Tansy
Foxglove (digitalis)	Wahoo
Hemlock	Wormwood
Jimsonweed	Yohimbe

THE CHINESE HERBAL PHARMACY

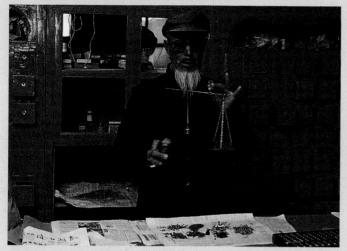

Chinese herbal medicine is thousands of years old, and many of the ideas developed in its infancy are still in use among practitioners throughout the world. For example, the prescriptions shown above, carved on wooden strips, are considered as effective today as when they were first created more than 2,000 years ago.

Throughout the ages, Chinese medical writings have expanded upon past wisdom. Thus, when Chang Chung-ching (A.D. 142-220), who is regarded as the Hippocrates of China, described 287 herbal formulas in his *Treatise on Febrile Diseases and Summaries of Household Remedies,* he drew many of his prescriptions from earlier dynasties. In turn, Chung's followers expanded upon his writings.

During the Ming dynasty (1368-1643), herbal medicine reached new heights—the famed *General Catalog of Herbs* by Li Shih-chen (1518-1593) describes 1,871 herbs and 8,160 herbal prescriptions. In China today, most people continue to rely on ancient herbal remedies, even though they may also see a physician who has been trained in Western medical practices.

Herbal Classification

Chinese herbalists stress that great care is needed to prevent mixing of drugs that are incompatible. Thus, herbal formulas are based upon very specific classifications according to their physical characteristics, and whether they are yin (cool or cold) or yang (warm or hot). More specifically, drugs are classified as follows:

▶ Five flavors: hot, which rid the body of toxins; sour, which are astringents or absorbents; sweet, which are tonics that reinforce warm drugs; bitter, which dry out and purge the body; and salty, which soften and lubricate.

▶ Four directions of action: ascending and floating, which are yang in nature and help expel or purge; and descending and sinking, which are yin in nature and move inward.

While under treatment, patients are also instructed to eat foods that are compatible with the yin or yang nature of their drugs.

Categories of Treatment

Chinese herbal treatments work by inducing one or more of the following physical responses:

▶ Sweating
▶ Vomiting
▶ Purging (promoting elimination via the colon)
▶ Harmonizing (restoring the body's natural homeostasis)
▶ Warming
▶ Removing
▶ Supplementing
▶ Reducing

Specific herbal remedies fall into 17 different categories:

▶ Anthelmintics to kill intestinal parasites.
▶ Antirheumatics, which are taken with sweating agents to treat rheumatism and arthritis.
▶ Antitussives and expectorants to treat coughs, asthma, and excess sputum production.
▶ Astringents to treat rectal prolapse, diarrhea, or sweating.
▶ Blood agents to treat anemia, menstrual problems, ulcers, and other disorders related to bleeding.
▶ Cold agents to treat colds, vomiting, diarrhea, and other symptoms.
▶ Digestive agents to treat abdominal pain and loss of appetite.
▶ Distress agents to treat psychological problems.
▶ Diuretics to treat edema and urinary problems.
▶ Emetics to treat chest congestion, intoxication, or overeating.
▶ External medicines, ointments, and sprays. These preparations are generally toxic if taken internally.
▶ Inhalants to treat fainting, unconsciousness, and high fevers.
▶ Purgatives to treat constipation.
▶ Refreshing agents to detoxify blood during a fever or infection.
▶ Sweating agents to treat such disorders as fevers and chills.
▶ Tonics to treat general weakness.
▶ Tranquilizers to reduce anxiety and treat insomnia and convulsions.

---

a DIN, Health Canada will accept the traditional claims for a medicinal herb, provided the claims are for self-diagnosable and self-treatable conditions and provided they are supported by two recognized authoritative herbal references.

Precautions

▶ Many plants are poisonous. Make sure that you know exactly what is in an herbal remedy before you take it internally.
▶ Before using any herbal remedy for a child's illness, consult a pediatrician or pediatric nurse.
▶ Take only the recommended dosage. Herbal products that are safe in small amounts can produce severe side effects when taken in larger doses. For example, a plant substance that may be an effective laxative in small quantities can often provoke severe diarrhea when taken in a larger dosage.
▶ Monitor yourself for possible side effects. If you develop a widespread rash, dizziness, difficulty breathing, or other signs of a severe reaction, call a doctor or go to your nearest emergency room because you may be having an anaphylactic reaction.

Labels should specify claims, dosage, caution, manner of preparation, and the quantity of the basic herb (crude or dried) per unit (tablet, teaspoon, milliliter) of the finished product.

What to expect

After asking questions about the nature of a problem, an herbalist will prescribe a specific plant and give instructions on how to use it. For medicinal purposes, dried herbs are usually recommended because their increased concentration makes them more potent than the fresh plants.

Leaves and flowers are dried in an airy, shady place; sun bakes out their oils and may also damage other medicinal ingredients. Roots and heavy stems are cleaned, chopped, dried, and then stored in glass jars or other nonmetallic containers in a cool, dry place until they are used.

Medicinal herbs are most often steeped in boiling water and consumed as a tea. These teas, which can be unpleasantly bitter or strong-tasting, should not be confused with the pleasant, commercially available herbal teas, which contain only a small fraction of the herbs used in a medicinal brew.

EXAMPLES OF COMMON HERBAL REMEDIES

Herb	Used for	Precautions
Aloe vera	Skin moisturizer; minor cuts; sunburn	Sometimes promoted as a laxative or for stomach disorders, but internal use is hazardous.
Anise	Cough soother; digestive aid	Generally safe.
Arnica	Anti-inflammatory painkiller for sprains, bruises; muscle aches	For external use only. Causes cardiac toxicity if ingested; stop using if arnica liniment causes dermatitis.
Buckthorn	Laxative; digestive aid; tonic; skin irritations	Generally safe in small doses. Should not be taken during pregnancy.
Chamomile	Tea: sedative; digestive aid; menstrual cramps. Compress: arthritis; skin disorders	Generally safe in small amounts.
Comfrey	Skin wounds, bruises, burns, and boils; reducing swelling of sprains; skin softener	Should not be taken internally because of possible liver toxicity.
Dandelion	Laxative; tonic; diuretic	Generally safe.
Echinacea	Compress: skin sores and stings. Tea: bladder infections; fever; headache	Generally safe in small doses.
Eucalyptus	Nasal and sinus congestion; coughs	Oil irritating to eyes and mucous membranes.
Evening primrose	Painkiller; sedative; autoimmune disorders	Can worsen bleeding disorders.
Fenugreek	Expectorant; digestive tonic; laxative. Poultice: Soothing of boils and skin ulcers	Generally safe.
Fennel	Digestive aid	Generally safe.
Feverfew	Painkiller	Generally safe; may cause mouth sores when chewed.
Garlic	Antiseptic; reducing of high blood pressure and high blood cholesterol	Generally safe, but raw garlic may irritate skin and mucous membranes; should not substitute for prescribed drugs.
Ginseng	General tonic; blood thinner; aphrodisiac	Generally safe, but many claims of its healing power are unproved.
Horehound	Decongestant; expectorant; cough soother; lowering of fever	Generally safe.
Hyssop	Expectorant, sore throat, coughs, digestive aid	Generally safe.
Licorice	Irritated skin and mucous membranes; ulcers; digestive aid	Generally safe; excessive use raises blood pressure.
Marshmallow	Demulcent to sooth intestinal inflammation and irritation; wound healing	Generally safe; excessive use may cause diarrhea.
Peppermint	Digestive aid	Generally safe.
Sassafras	Skin wounds; relief of poison ivy rash	Should not be taken internally.
Uva-ursi	Diuretic; cystitis; kidney and bladder stones	Generally safe, but should not substitute for antibiotics.
Valerian	Sleep aid; relieving of stress	Generally safe, but should not be used during pregnancy.
Witch hazel	Astringent; skin irritations; hemorrhoids	Should not be taken internally.

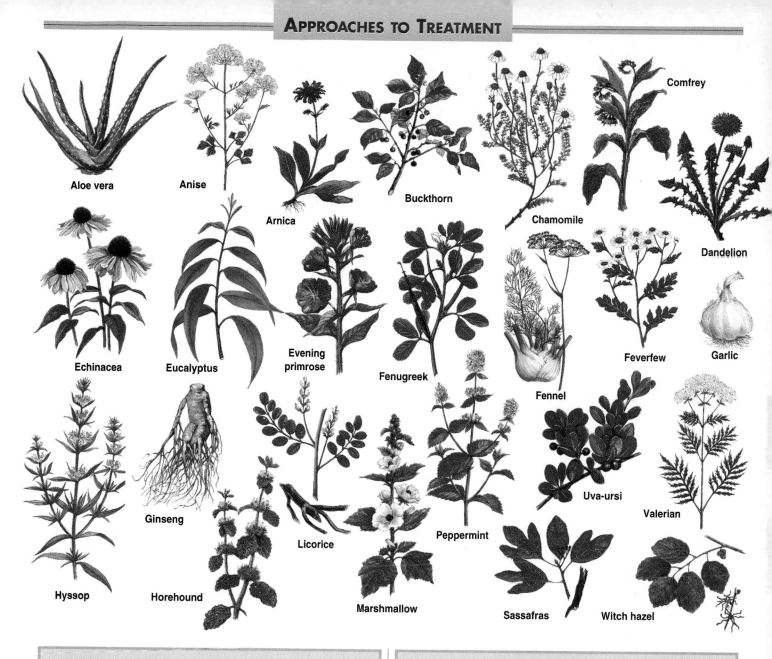

Aloe vera

Anise

Arnica

Buckthorn

Chamomile

Comfrey

Dandelion

Echinacea

Eucalyptus

Evening primrose

Fenugreek

Fennel

Feverfew

Garlic

Ginseng

Licorice

Peppermint

Uva-ursi

Valerian

Hyssop

Horehound

Marshmallow

Sassafras

Witch hazel

HERBAL RECIPES

Herbal preparations are taken in many forms—alcohol tinctures, fluid extracts, essential oils, syrups, vinegars, capsules, and pills. Lay people are generally advised to obtain these preparations from reliable herbalists or reputable commercial outlets. If you prefer to make your own, herbalists recommend freshly made infusions (teas) or decoctions using the following recipes:

Standard infusion. Place 1 ounce of dried herb or 3 ounces of fresh herb in a teapot or other nonmetalic container, and pour in 1 pint of boiling water. Let it steep for 10 minutes, strain out herbs, and drink while still fresh. (Note: Some remedies may call for stronger or milder teas; adjust recipe according to instructions.)

Decoction. Place 1 ounce of herb in a glass, enamel, or stainless steel pan (not aluminum), add 3 cups of water and bring to a boil; lower heat and simmer for 10 minutes or until the liquid is reduced by one-third. Strain and drink the recommended amount while the liquid is still hot. (Note: decoctions are usually made from roots or woody herbs.)

Compresses. Soak gauze or fine cloth in an infusion or decoction and apply to skin. (Test first on a small area for irritation.)

Poultice. Boil or cook herb (for example, garlic) or other recommended substance (for example, oatmeal), wrap in gauze, press out excess fluid, and apply while still hot.

BACH FLOWER REMEDIES

Of the several variations on herbalism, one of the best known is the system of Dr. Edward Bach (1886-1936), an English bacteriologist and homeopath who created and used flower essences as an alternative to conventional drug remedies. His preparations were made by immersing flowers in water and then exposing this combination to heat or to sunlight.

Afterward, the plants are discarded and the water is preserved in brandy. Bach believed that flower essences, individually and in combination, would restore the mental and emotional balance essential for physical well-being.

The best-known of the Bach concoctions is the Rescue Remedy, a combination of five different formulas, which is reserved for sudden trauma (brought on by bad news, for example), as well as episodes of panic, anxiety, or dread. Other Bach remedies include agrimony to relieve anxiety, impatiens to reduce emotional irritability; and a combination of larch, holly, and mustard flower essences for asthma.

Flower essences are sold in small bottles with eye droppers from which a drop or two is usually placed under the tongue at specified times. The drops are sold at some health food stores and pharmacies, or by mail order from England (many of the flower species are found only there).

Homeopathy

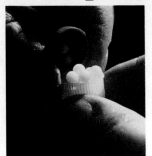

Homeopathic medicines are so diluted that only an undetectable fraction remains.

Homeopathy is based on the theory that the cause of an illness is similar to its cure. Thus, treatment involves giving a small amount of a very diluted natural substance that, if taken in larger doses, would cause the same symptoms as the ailment itself.

Origins

Samuel Hahnemann, a German physician, evolved the principles of homeopathy early in the 19th century, after abandoning what he considered to be the crude practices of his colleagues. He became especially interested in references to "similars" by Paracelsus, a 16th-century Swiss physician and alchemist who had concluded that the same substances which cause illness in large amounts will cure it in small doses. After conducting experiments, Hahnemann announced his findings in 1810, and a list of "proven" remedies appeared in 1821. Hahnemann's principles of homeopathy state that:

▶ Substances that produce symptoms similar or identical to those experienced by the patient will produce the cure; in other words, "like cures like."

▶ Only one medicine is given at a time.

▶ The least possible amount of the curative substance is the most effective for relieving symptoms.

▶ The patient's positive attitude is an essential factor in the success of the healing process.

Homeopathic practice became the rage in Europe and North America and, in 1844, the American Institute of Homeopathy was established by a group of distinguished doctors. When the American Medical Association was founded a few years later, it took a hostile position against its predecessor. In a short time, homeopathy declined in the United States, but it never went out of style in Europe. Homeopathic pharmacies, hospitals, and clinics abound throughout Europe

Precautions

▶ Beware of extravagant claims by any practitioner who holds out the promise of a cure for a serious condition that is unresponsive to conventional treatment.

▶ If your symptoms haven't been alleviated in one or two homeopathic visits, it's time to see your physician.

▶ A large number of homeopathic guides and remedies can be found in health food stores. Such self-treatment should be confined to minor ailments.

today, and the services are covered by most national health insurance plans.

In North America, homeopathy is enjoying a revival, because its adherents consider it a natural approach and its treatments do not cause the side effects of many of the drugs used in conventional medicine.

Practitioners

According to the Ontario Homeopathic Association, there are some 200 homeopaths in Canada, about half of them are physicians. Because homeopathy is not regulated, Canadian homeopaths need no accreditation. Homeopathic preparations have been legal in Canada since the 1980s.

When it is used

Homeopaths claim to treat virtually all conditions, but most concede that their methods work best against chronic disorders such as headaches, allergies, intestinal diseases, and asthma. Remedies are often prescribed as an adjunct to other alternative procedures, such as acupuncture and chiropractic. Most homeopaths recommend that conventional medicine also be used for injuries, infections, and cancer and other serious diseases. In these cases, homeopathy is considered an adjunct to enhance the effect of conventional medicine.

How it works

Even the most enthusiastic proponents of homeopathy are not sure exactly how it works. Practitioners believe that symptoms are an expression of the body's attempt to heal itself. Therefore, they seek the substance that produces in healthy people the symptoms experienced in the illness.

Homeopathic medicines are prepared by a series of dilutions. An extract is mixed with 100 times as much water or water and alcohol, shaken energetically, then diluted again. Shaking between each dilution is essential; substances that are diluted without the shaking do not work. This process is repeated until it is impossible to discover any trace of the original extract.

Practitioners claim that the more diluted the remedy, the more effective it will be. They ascribe its effectiveness to the transmission of "vital energy" that resonates within the patient's body. Some assume that confidence in the healer can also improve the patient's condition.

What to expect

In the first encounter, a practitioner will ask many questions and conduct a physical examination. A single remedy is then selected. (Even if this treatment does not produce a cure, it is not likely to do any harm because it is so diluted.) If the wrong remedy is chosen, it is said to have missed the ailment's "center of gravity," and a different one will be tried. The correct remedy may worsen symptoms initially, indicating that the body's defenses are rallying to produce a cure.

THE MATERIA MEDICA OF HOMEOPATHY

Many homeopathic remedies are classified according to the symptoms that they are said to counter. Examples include:

▶ Aconite (monkshood). Symptoms, such as a high fever, are intense and come on suddenly. Aconite is normally administered at the onset of an illness.

▶ Apis Mellifica (honey bee venom). Symptoms include acute inflammation marked by stinging, burning, redness, and swelling.

▶ Arsenicum Album (white arsenic or arsenious acid). Symptoms include extreme agitation, fear, weakness, fatigue, chills, and burning pain, all worsening at night.

▶ Belladonna (deadly nightshade). Symptoms come on suddenly and violently, and may include fever, inflammation, and cramps.

▶ Gelsemium (yellow jasmine). Drowsiness, fatigue, mental sluggishness, and physical weakness predominate.

▶ Mercurius Vivus (mercury). Symptoms include marked inflammation of the skin and mucous membranes, pus formation, pain and, in some cases, open sores.

▶ Nux vomica (poison nut tree). Symptoms include headaches, chills, indigestion, muscle spasms, and back pain.

Hydrotherapy

Hydrotherapy is the use of water to treat disease, alleviate pain, induce relaxation, and maintain general good health. For therapeutic purposes, the water may be hot or cold, or in the form of ice or steam. Treatments include immersion baths (usually in cool water), hot tub soaks, sitz baths (a shortened hip bath), mud baths, steam baths, saunas, needle showers, salt rubs, pressure hosing, hot or cold packs, douches, and colonic irrigation (washing of the inner wall of the large intestine). Hydrotherapy may also take the form of drinking water that has special qualities, such as the mineral waters offered by European spas as an aid to digestion.

Origins
Because of the almost universal availability of water, it has been used to promote health and to cure illness by all cultures. The elaborate and efficient public baths built by the ancient Romans are a typical example; they were usually combined with gymnasiums to foster socializing and physical and mental well-being by alternating exercise with relaxation. In Finland, saunas have been a ritual for 2,000 years. Russian and Turkish steam baths, introduced years ago to North America by immigrant populations, remain popular to this day. In recent years, hydrotherapy has gained an important place in physical therapy and rehabilitation medicine.

Practitioners
In hospitals, hydrotherapy is performed by doctors, nurses, nurses' aides, and physical therapists. At a spa or health club, it may be supervised by a physical therapist, a massage specialist, or an ayurvedic practitioner. However, the most common site for hydrotherapy is the home, where the techniques are used as forms of self-treatment.

When it is used
In rehabilitation facilities and mental hospitals, hydrotherapy is used to relax muscles and joints, soothe anxiety, relieve stress, and enhance mobility. This last may be achieved through swimming and underwater exercise, which can help maintain and extend range of motion for patients who have arthritis and other joint and muscle disorders.

As part of a pain management program, hydrotherapy in the form of warm baths in a darkened room can help patients focus on breathing exercises and other pain-control methods.

Hydrotherapy is also promoted by health clubs and spas as a natural way of treating aching muscles and painful joints, with a combination of showers and steam or whirlpools, after participation in athletic activities.

At home, it is employed as an aid to relaxation, to alleviate minor aches and pains, and to induce sleep.

How it works
The way in which hydrotherapy works depends on its form:
▶ Sitz baths soothe many conditions, including hemorrhoids, anal fissures, and vaginal infections.

Precautions
▶ Pregnant women and people who have diabetes, high blood pressure, or any chronic coronary condition should avoid hot tubs, steam baths, and saunas.
▶ An ice pack should not be placed directly on the skin; instead, it should be wrapped in a towel or cloth.

WATER AEROBICS
An increasingly popular form of hydrotherapy is water aerobics, or modified aerobic dancing done in the shallow end of a swimming pool. Water aerobics offers all the benefits of other forms of aerobic exercise without the joint strain and risk of injury inherent in any weight-bearing activity. It is particularly beneficial for older people, pregnant women, anyone with a sports injury or arthritis, and those who are overweight.

▶ Floating in a pool or special tub permits a person who has arthritis or has suffered a stroke to exercise joints in a way that might otherwise be too difficult or painful.
▶ Medicinal baths in warm to hot water affect metabolism of the body tissues lying just under the skin, or improve circulation by increasing the flow of blood to surface areas.
▶ A steam bath clears nasal congestion and soothes sore muscles and stiff joints.
▶ An ice pack reduces swelling and inflammation following a bruise, sports injury, or tooth extraction.
▶ Medicated vapor relieves chest congestion.
▶ A warm, wet dressing helps to bring a boil to a head so that it can break on its own or be drained.
▶ Cold, wet towels wrapped around an individual suffering from heat exhaustion quickly bring down the person's temperature, and therefore are an effective emergency treatment.

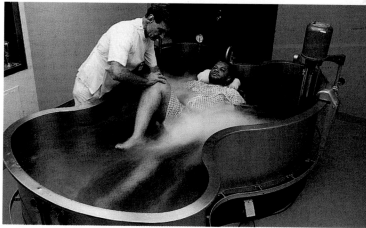

Underwater exercise is an important part of the physical therapy and rehabilitation of patients who have suffered a stroke or whose arthritis makes movement difficult and painful.

What to expect
In rehabilitation centers, hydrotherapy may include immersion baths, needle showers, underwater muscle massage with powerful water jets, douches, and cold or hot wet wrappings of a body part or of the entire body.

In the past, some forms of hydrotherapy were widely used to calm agitated or aggressive patients with mental illnesses. Today, medications have made this use of hydrotherapy largely obsolete. However, some mental institutions may employ a flotation tank to calm severely agitated patients. Use of such a tank induces deep relaxation by allowing the body to float in warm water, often in a darkened room from which all environmental stimuli have been removed.

Hypnosis

Hypnosis is an altered state of consciousness in which a very highly concentrated state of attention is focused on a specific idea or memory. The patient (or subject) is fully awake but responds only to the therapist's suggestions. There is abundant empirical evidence that hypnotherapy produces desired results for many people. Some, however, are incapable of achieving a deep trance state. Others can reach only a light hypnotic state because they are unable or unconsciously unwilling to achieve this form of total concentration.

Origins
From ancient healers to Dr. Franz Mesmer, an 18th-century Viennese physician who cast his subjects into a trance as a theatrical entertainment (hence mesmerizing), hypnosis has had a colorful history. Not until the late 1950s did it begin to

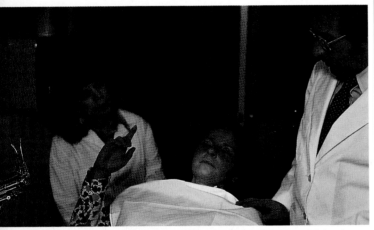

Hypnosis may be a solution for a dental patient who cannot tolerate anesthesia or one who has an intense fear of dental procedures.

overcome its association with charlatans and movie villains. Today, hypnosis is recognized by the medical community in North America as a useful therapeutic tool.

Practitioners
Hypnotherapy, as the medical use of hypnosis is called, is practiced by physicians (especially psychiatrists), dentists, psychologists, naturopaths, physical therapists, psychiatric social workers, and holistic healers. Legitimate hypnotherapy should not be confused with staged hypnosis, which is sometimes presented as entertainment.

When it is used
A psychotherapist or other health-care professional may use hypnosis in several ways. One is behavior modification; for example, helping a patient to overcome a weight problem or nicotine addiction. Another is the calling up of traumatic events, such as childhood abuse, that may have been denied

---

Precautions
▶ Be wary of self-styled hynotherapists who advertise their services in the Yellow Pages or newspaper classified ads. Instead, ask your doctor for a referral or call the psychiatry department of the nearest teaching hospital and ask for names of qualified hypnotherapists in your area.

VISUALIZATION
Visualization entails concentrating fully on a specific image. It may be combined with hypnosis or another therapy to induce relaxation, counteract anxiety, or control pain perception.

Dr. Herbert Benson, a Harvard psychologist and author of *The Relaxation Response,* urges patients to use visualization to overcome stress. For example, he instructs them to visualize a peaceful landscape while tensing and relaxing different muscle groups to achieve more complete relaxation.

---

or buried as a means of self-protection. Two other uses are the diagnosing of multiple personalities and the treating of phobias, such as fear of flying.

Pain management is another major application of hypnosis. A deep trance state may be induced to serve as anesthesia during surgery; a lighter trance is often employed to ease the pain of childbirth. And for controlling chronic pain, many people are now taught the techniques of self-hypnosis.

How it works
To control pain through hypnosis, patients are taught to become intensely aware of their body sensations, to track their breathing, and to eliminate distracting thoughts and images. Then they are instructed to focus on the pain—its location, intensity, and shape. Through this technique, they become active participants in pain control, learning to modify its features, shift its level, and raise and lower its intensity. Eventually they can learn to transfer the skills developed during hypnosis to control other troublesome problems.

To help a patient remember a blocked out traumatic event or a critical childhood experience, the hypnotist will put him in a hypnotic trance and suggest mentally going back to the time and place in question. This regression is often done in steps; for example, he may be instructed to visit a childhood classroom or former home. Typically, the subject begins to speak in a childlike voice and assume a different posture. If the flashback scene is especially painful, he may cry, but the crying is likely to be that of a child, rather than an adult. After the subject is instructed to end the trance, voice and posture return to normal, and often there is no memory of what happened during hypnosis.

In diagnosing and treating multiple personality disorders, the hypnotist tries to get the other personalities to come forth. Again, there is often a dramatic change in voice and bearing as different personalities emerge.

What to expect
A hypnotic trance is most successfully induced in a subject who is cooperative and who can relax, maintain a state of mental alertness, and concentrate on repeated instructions, which sometimes involve visualization (see box, above). They may be repeated in a low, confident voice as the hypnotherapist leads the subject into a deep trance. As the suggestibility level increases, breathing and pulse rate slow down. At this point, the therapist can instill desired images; for example, having a smoker concentrate on a scenario in which all ashtrays are discarded and all tobacco smoke becomes noxious.

Most patients can learn the techniques of self-hypnosis and visualization, thereby reinforcing and extending the efforts of the therapist. Audio and video tapes that offer instructions in hypnosis and visualization are available for home use.

Light Therapy

Light therapy employs either natural or artificial light to treat various disorders, ranging from psoriasis and other skin diseases to soft bones and seasonal affective disorder (SAD), a type of depression that occurs during the winter.

Origins

Exposure to bright sunlight and to the ultraviolet rays of sun lamps has been used to treat skin diseases for many years. The application of light therapy for treating SAD dates from the late 1980s when doctors first recognized the link between depression and the long, dark days of mid-winter.

Practitioners

Light therapy may be administered by psychiatrists, general practitioners, or their assistants. It can also be carried out at home under instructions by a qualified health professional.

When it is used

Light therapy is now the treatment of choice for SAD, largely replacing the use of antidepressants and psychotherapy.

Ultraviolet light has several uses. One is to treat psoriasis, often in conjunction with drugs, as well as other nonspecific skin conditions that cause itching. Another is to treat rickets

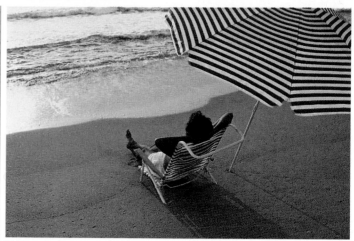

Taking a winter vacation in a warm, sunny clime is a good way to beat the winter blues, but one should be careful not to indulge in too much direct sun exposure, which can damage the skin.

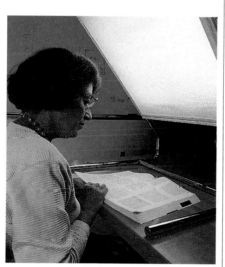

While underoing light therapy, a patient can read or go about other routine activities that can be done while sitting.

(in children) or osteomalacia (in adults). These disorders, in which the bones become soft, are caused by a lack of vitamin D, which the body makes when the skin is exposed to sunlight. Elderly shut-ins benefit from such treatment in two ways: The light therapy helps strengthen their bones, and at the same time helps them counter depression. Infants born with jaundice are also sometimes exposed to ultraviolet light.

Precautions

▶ Light therapy is effective only with lights specifically designed for this purpose. Other types of bright lights, such as halogen lamps and sunlamps, are not suitable.
▶ To avoid eye irritation and damage, do not look directly at the light source. Always cover the eyes of babies who are being exposed to bright, direct light.
▶ Because ultraviolet light increases the risk of skin cancer, its use should be carefully monitored by a doctor.

Other potential uses of light therapy include treatment for jet lag, sleep disorders, and the biorhythm problems that are often experienced by people who work at night.

How it works

Exposure to varying levels of light affects the biological clock of all living creatures. In humans, lack of sunshine has a more profound psychological effect than was formerly recognized. (Some researchers estimate that 20 percent of people who live in the northern United States and Canada could benefit from light therapy, with women outnumbering men four to one.) Daylight stimulates the human brain to produce hormones and other brain chemicals that are essential for psychological and emotional well-being.

For most SAD sufferers, daily exposure to a few hours of very bright fluorescent lights relieves their symptoms as effectively as a winter vacation in the sunny tropics. Within four days of beginning treatment, most patients show a marked improvement—much more quickly than with antidepressant medication. Benefits seem to be the same whether therapy takes place during the day or night.

Ultraviolet light also directly affects the skin in several ways: It promotes the manufacture of vitamin D and slows the growth of new skin cells in psoriasis. Its drying effect may help improve acne. In some people, however, sunlight triggers a flare-up of acne; one should proceed with caution.

What to expect

The special fluorescent lights used for treating SAD are housed in boxes containing a reflector and a light-diffusing cover. The treatments, which are simple, painless, inexpensive, and harmless when done properly, usually take two or three hours a day, although some people benefit from as little as half an hour of exposure.

During a treatment, the patient can nap, read, or go about other quiet activities. New types of light therapy devices that would not interfere with a patient's daily routine are being investigated. One of these is a computer-controlled gadget that switches on a bright light early in the morning to simulate the arrival of dawn before the time of the usual winter sunrise. Studies at New York's Columbia-Presbyterian Medical Center, where the device was developed, found that test volunteers woke up feeling alert and vigorous.

Macrobiotics

Macrobiotics is a dietary discipline based on the East Asian concept that good health depends on establishing a harmonious balance of the opposing life forces (yang and yin), and that this applies to foods as well as other aspects of life.

Origins

The regimen was developed during the first half of the 20th century by George Ohsawa, a Japanese philosophy student who claimed to have cured his tuberculosis by devising a diet based on the spiritual principles and practices of Oriental medicine. He created the term macrobiotics, which in Greek means "a broad view of life," and described his regimen in a 1920 book, *A New Theory of Nutrition and Its Therapeutic Effect*. The book is now in its 700th edition in Japan.

By the time of his death in 1966, Ohsawa had written over 300 books and had traveled throughout the world promoting his dietary philosophy. He found a receptive audience in the early 1960s among young North Americans, who flocked to macrobiotic restaurants and health food stores.

Practitioners

A number of alternative therapists, including acupuncturists, naturopaths, practitioners of Oriental medicine, and holistic healers, have incorporated macrobiotics into their practices.

When it is used

As a therapy, macrobiotics is used to treat various ailments through a limited diet. It may, for example, be recommended as a treatment for eating disorders or for coping with stress. Many of its proponents also believe that it provides a spiritual or mystical foundation for the way life should be lived.

How it works

Macrobiotics classifies all foods as yang or yin instead of by nutritional content and the designations of carbohydrate, protein, and fat (see box, below). In general, a macrobiotic

IS IT YIN OR YANG? The macrobiotic classification of foods as yin or yang weighs at least 15 factors. Plant foods are generally yin, representing the earth's upward force. Thus, they are thought to slow metabolism, have a calming effect, and produce other yin effects, such as reducing body temperature. Animal foods represent the heaven's downward, or yang, force, and have the opposite effect of speeding up metabolism.

Within each classification, however, there are many gradations, ranging from most yin to most yang (see box, below left).

Geography and the season are also taken into consideration. As much as possible, foods should be locally grown. Persons who live in cold, northern (yin) climates should lean toward yang foods and means of preparation, while the opposite applies to those living in warmer (yang) climates. Similarly, yin foods and cooking methods are to be followed during the warm summer months, and yang foods and preparation should dominate in the colder winter months.

diet calls for 50 to 60 percent of calories to come from whole cereal grains, the foods that are most balanced in yin and yang; 25 to 30 percent from vegetables; 10 to 15 percent from beans and sea vegetables; 5 to 10 percent from fish, shellfish, seasonal fruits, and nuts; and 5 percent from soups made with vegetables, grains, or miso (fermented soy).

The extreme macrobiotic diets of the early 1960s were sometimes limited to brown rice only, which is balanced in its yin and yang qualities but is not complete nutritionally. Those were soon abandoned when faithful followers developed severe malnutrition. Today's macrobiotic diet is similar to many vegetarian regimens, especially those that eschew milk and eggs but allow inclusion of seafood.

What to expect

Following a diagnosis based on the individual's appearance, symptoms, and current diet, the macrobiotic therapist recommends changes aimed at correcting the imbalance of yang and yin foods. Modifications depend on the availability of local grains, vegetables, and fruit. Brown rice and herbal tea are considered basic. Bananas, mangoes, and other tropical fruits are avoided in temperate climates. Even though fish and some meat may be acceptable, all dairy products are excluded. Processed foods, whether frozen or canned, are also prohibited at all times.

A person may be taught new ways in which to prepare foods. Copper and aluminum pans, for example, are not used because traces of their metals can leach into foods. Instead, stainless steel, enamel, glass, and ceramic cookware, as well as wooden or bamboo spoons, are recommended.

MACROBIOTIC FOOD CLASSIFICATION

Food group	More Yin	More Yang
Grains	Corn, long-grain rice, summer wheat	Millet, buckwheat, short-grain rice, winter wheat
Beans	Soybeans and other oily beans	Chickpeas, lentils, and other nonoily beans
Vegetables	All those grown above ground	Carrots and other root vegetables
Seaweed	Harvested in warm water close to shore	Harvested in deeper, cold water
Nuts	Peanuts, cashews, and other oily nuts	Almonds, chestnuts, and other less oily nuts
Fruits	Citrus, mango, and other tropical fruits	Apples, cherries, and other temperate fruits
Sweetners	Sugar, honey, and maple syrup	Barley malt and rice honey

Precautions

▶A rigorous macrobiotic diet can have dangerous consequences if imposed on children and adolescents. Because it is low in calories and certain nutrients, it can also further jeopardize the health of people with AIDS, cancer, and malabsorption diseases.
▶ If you devise your own macrobiotic diet as a way of losing weight, ask your doctor or a qualified nutritionist about supplements, especially of vitamin B_{12}.

Massage

In therapeutic massage, touch is used to induce relaxation and promote well-being. Though there are many forms of the practice, all employ systematic stroking, rubbing, pressing, kneading, or thumping of the skin, muscles, and joints. Massage is also combined sometimes with other techniques, especially aroma and water therapies.

Origins

Massage is an instinctive means of communication and giving comfort. Among animals, mothers stroke their young, and the adults of many species rub or groom each other.

Medically, massage is our oldest form of treatment and one that is used by every culture. The earliest Chinese, Egyptian, and Indian medical writings all describe preventive and ther-

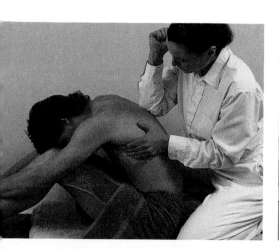

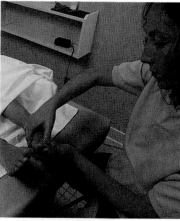

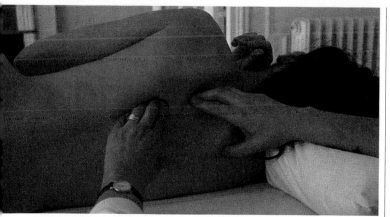

Rolfing (upper left) involves pummeling and deep massage to manipulate connective tissue. In contrast, reflexology (upper right) concentrates on stimulating specific pressure points, usually on the feet. Shiatsu (lower photo) is another form of pressure-point massage.

apeutic uses of massage. Galen, a second-century Roman physician, massaged both the emperor and gladiators, and wrote more than a dozen medical books about massage.

The most familiar form in North America, Swedish, or classic massage, was developed in Sweden in the early 1800s by Per Henrik Ling; before his death in 1838, institutes for it had been established in several countries.

Following World War I, massage by hand was gradually replaced by the electrical devices used in physical therapy. By the 1940s, massage therapy had been eclipsed by modern

medicine, and it was relegated to seedy massage parlors or scorned as a pleasure of the pampered rich. In recent years, the pendulum has begun to swing back, and massage by hand is once again considered a useful therapeutic tool.

Practitioners

Almost everyone can do a simple form of massage on himself or someone else, but special instruction is needed to master the techniques of the specific therapeutic form. In Canada, training in Swedish massage varies from province to province. For example, the College of Massage Therapists of Ontario in Toronto requires 2,200 hours of study, including courses in anatomy and physiology. There are also institutes that teach and certify other specialized forms of massage such as reflexology and shiatsu, techniques in which specific pressure points are pressed or massaged to alleviate pain and other symptoms.

Most massage therapists practice independently, although some work in tandem with physical therapists, sports medicine physicians, rehabilitation specialists, osteopaths, chiropractors, and other health professionals. To find a reputable practitioner, call the rehabilitation, or physiatry, department of a hospital.

When it is used

Massage is employed to alleviate stiffness, tension, and soreness in muscles, and to promote comfort and help overcome stress. Many athletic trainers recommend massage to loosen muscles before competition as well as to ease soreness afterwards. Massage can also relieve leg cramps. If you are often awakened by leg cramps or suffer restless leg syndrome, try massaging your legs before going to bed. Back and shoulder massages help some women manage labor pains, and gentle massage is one way to comfort a colicky baby. Migraines and tension headaches can be alleviated by massage; the same is true of lower back pain due to muscle spasms.

How it works

In general, massage works by easing muscle and psychological tension and promoting relaxation. The use of aromatic oils during massage—a variation of aromatherapy—can help deepen relaxation. Massage increases blood flow to the area being rubbed, and this may speed healing. Contrary to common claims, however, massage cannot speed the expelling of toxins from the body.

Practitioners of massage techniques that employ pressure points—for example, shiatsu, reflexology, and acupressure—claim benefits similar to those of acupuncture. The idea is to apply pressure to a specific part of the body to elicit a response elsewhere (see next page for more details.)

What to expect

For Swedish, or European, massage, the person receiving treatment undresses and then reclines on a padded table, mattress, or floor pad, and the massager stands or kneels at his side. A towel or sheet is draped over parts of the body that are not being massaged. A warm, often scented oil is applied to the exposed skin, which is then massaged with different strokes. Depending upon the stroke, the fingers, thumbs, palms, or edges of the hand, as well as elbows and forearms, are used. Most strokes are gentle and pleasant. In deep massage, however, the muscles are vigorously prodded

MASSAGE (CONTINUED)

and thumped. The effect should be invigorating rather than uncomfortable; let the practitioner know if the massage produces any sharp or radiating pain.

Rolfing, another vigorous form of massage, involves manipulating the deep connective tissue, or fascia, that holds the muscles together. During a session, the rolfer uses his hands, fingers, and elbows to press deeply or pummel different parts of the body. A session can be quite painful, but devotees say they feel wonderful afterwards.

There are a few other therapies that incorporate massage as part of their overall approach. For example, Hellerwork, an outgrowth of rolfing, combines deep-tissue massage with posture exercises. And polarity uses massage to harness and redirect the body's flow of energy. It also employs yoga, exercise, and nutritional and psychological counseling to provide a total approach to health and healing.

Precautions

▶ Refrain from massage during a fever, infectious illness, or bout of phlebitis, because it may worsen the underlying condition.
▶ Avoid rolfing and other deep-tissue massage techniques if you have osteoporosis or similar bone disorders; vigorous pummeling may result in a fracture.
▶ Discontinue back massage immediately if it produces a sharp pain or sends pain radiating to the buttocks or legs.
▶ Avoid massaging directly over a bruise, burn, unhealed wound or incision, varicose vein, or skin infection or rash. Instead, gently massage the adjacent areas to ease discomfort.
▶ Consult your doctor before undergoing massage if you have a chronic disorder such as diabetes or heart disease.
▶ Steer clear of massagers who advertise their services in the personal columns, especially those offering sensuous massages.

PRESSURE-POINT MASSAGE TECHNIQUES

Shiatsu, acupressure, zone therapy, and other pressure-point massage techniques differ from whole-body massage in that they concentrate on specific points, which are comparable to the acupoints of acupuncture. The objective is to maintain or restore the proper flow and balance of vital energy within the body.

Shiatsu. This is a Japanese massage technique that combines aspects of Chinese acupuncture and philosophy with body massage. Pressure points, or tsubos, are situated along 12 pathways, or meridians, extending from head to toe or fingertip. Shiatsu practitioners believe that the life energy, or qi, flows along these meridians; pain and disease occur when this energy flow is blocked or misdirected.

The area between the ribs and pelvis, referred to as the hara, is considered the body's storehouse of qi, and a shiatsu treatment begins and ends with the therapist massaging this section. A proper flow of energy is then restored by massaging and pressing upon the relevant tsubos.

Practitioners also strive to bring the force of yin, which is deep and internal, and yang, which is more active and superficial, into proper harmony. Thus, a patient suffering from yin symptoms such as fatigue and drowsiness would be given a treatment designed to stimulate the more energetic yang forces, whereas a calming yin treatment would be admin-istered to a person complaining of headache or restlessness.

During a typical shiatsu session, the person may be clothed or unclothed and usually lies on a carpeted floor or mat, with the therapist kneeling at her side. Pressure is applied mostly with the fingers, although practitioners may also use the entire hand, elbow, knee, and other body parts. A session lasts generally from 45 to 60 minutes,

and the areas being massaged may vary depending upon whether there is an underlying disorder. Although shiatsu is used to treat certain medical problems, such as back pain or headaches, it is more often considered a preventive therapy to help keep the body functioning properly.

Acupressure. This technique differs from shiatsu in that its goal is to treat specific disorders by pressing upon the acupoints

Pressure Points in Reflexology

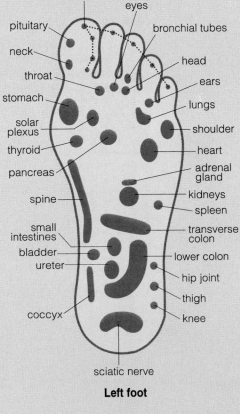

sinuses
eyes
pituitary
bronchial tubes
neck
throat
head
ears
stomach
lungs
solar plexus
shoulder
thyroid
heart
pancreas
adrenal gland
spine
kidneys
spleen
small intestines
transverse colon
bladder
ureter
lower colon
hip joint
thigh
coccyx
knee

sciatic nerve

Left foot

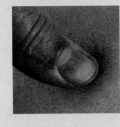

Reflexologists stimulate specific points on the foot or hand to treat disorders of corresponding internal organs. The objective is to redirect the flow of the body's bioelectrical energy.

used by acupuncturists. The appropriate acupoint is identified, and the therapist uses a fingertip or thumb to press upon it. A circular motion may then be used to stimulate deep, constant pressure.

Reflexology. Also referred to as zone therapy, reflexology aims to treat disorders by massaging and stimulating points, usually on the hands and feet, that correspond to specific internal organs. Unlike acupressure and shiatsu, which originated in Asia, reflexology was developed by an American, Dr. William Fitzgerald, an ear, nose, and throat specialist who introduced the technique in 1913.

Fitzgerald divided the body into 10 vertical zones through which he believed bioelectrical energy flowed to specific points in the hands and feet. In the 1940s, Eunice Ingham, a physical therapist, refined Fitzgerald's techniques, concentrating on pressure points in the feet. Today, reflexologists may use points in the feet, hands, ears, and elsewhere on the body, although foot massage remains the primary focus of the discipline. The basic techniques are finger walking, in which fingers are inched over the foot by bending and unbending the first joint; flexing, in which a thumb is pressed into the sole and the foot is then flexed several times; thumb walking, in which the thumb is inched up the sole of the foot toward the toes; and finger rolling, in which the tip of each toe is massaged with the tip of the index finger.

Meditation

Meditation is a mental discipline that is aimed at achieving complete relaxation. It is often promoted as an alternative to tranquilizers and painkillers in the management of emotional stress and physical pain.

Origins

This ancient art has been used for centuries by both healers and spiritual leaders. It is a central practice in many Eastern religions. Buddhist spiritual leaders, for example, believe that meditation frees the mind to release its healing power. In North America, widespread interest in meditation dates to the 1960s when Maharishi Mahesh Yogi came from India to teach his technique. Known as transcendental meditation, it is based on an ancient Indian system, adapted for Western use. It requires no special mental or physical discipline other than the chanting of, or concentration on, a specific sound or thought during two daily half-hour sessions. By the early 1970s, some 90,000 men and women had tried this form of meditation, and many of them volunteered as subjects of medical studies to document its effects. Today, there are centers for transcendental meditation in Toronto, Montreal, Vancouver, and other large Canadian centers.

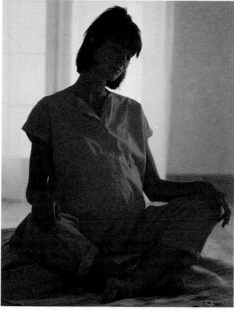

Some childbirth educators teach meditation as a way to overcome fear and manage pain.

Practitioners

Classes in meditation are sometimes conducted by physicians, psychologists, and physical therapists, as well as by yoga instructors, acupuncturists, and other alternative practitioners. Therapists trained in the techniques have been conducting classes in schools of the performing arts, and they are being invited into the corporate world to teach meditation for stress management. Some have also put their instructions on tapes and in books for home use.

When it is used

Meditation is used as a means of managing pain, coping with psychological stress, overcoming insomnia, and dealing with panic and anxiety. It is also an adjunct to conventional medicine in controlling asthma, high blood pressure, angina, and other chronic disorders.

How it works

Research indicates that meditation produces changes in the nervous system that are the opposite of the "fight-or-flight" response to danger. Specifically, meditation appears to reduce the body's production of cortisol, the hormone that triggers the response. Reduced cortisol levels foster relaxation.

Western researchers, who have studied the physical effects of meditation on yogis and Zen Buddhists as they are in the process of using it, have found that it slows metabolism, reduces oxygen consumption, and lowers carbon dioxide production. Brain studies done in the United States and in Japan indicate that there is also an increase in alpha brain waves, which normally occur during relaxation.

What to expect

As the aim of meditation is to achieve a heightened sense of mindfulness through concentration, activities are geared to this goal. For example, Dr. Jon Kabat-Zinn, a psychologist who pioneered the use of meditation in pain management, starts by urging members of a group to concentrate totally on each detail of a raisin: its appearance, feel, smell, taste, texture, and so on. Participants are then asked to transfer this heightened awareness to their breathing. Finally, they are instructed to focus completely on their pain, so they can begin to gain control over it.

The ability to concentrate on breathing to the exclusion of all other activities also has a calming effect, which can help overcome anxiety and relieve panic attacks. By focusing entirely on taking in and letting out one deep breath at a time, a person can control the feelings of panic.

Precautions

▶ If you're experiencing pain or other distressing symptoms, consult a doctor for a diagnosis before you join a meditation group.

▶ Although meditation lowers blood pressure, the effect is usually temporary. Hence, the technique should be used in conjunction with, not as a substitute for, conventional hypertension therapy.

HEALING IMAGES

Guided imagery, also referred to as waking dream therapy, uses mental pictures to fight disease and produce other desired effects. Until recently, imagery was practiced mostly by psychiatrists. A celebrated example was the 14-year-old boy whose tic was permanently cured by Sigmund Freud through imagery—the only complete cure described in all of Freud's case studies, and the only one in which he used this method.

Today, both alternative and conventional health professionals are teaching imagery to patients who have a variety of ailments, everything from stress-related headaches to cancer. In simple terms, imagery attempts to enlist the brain to play an active part in healing. For example, the Simonton Imagery Process encourages cancer patients to imagine the positive effects of radiation on cancer cells, and to enjoy the feeling of control that comes from being in touch with the body. It is thought that this psychological involvement strengthens the patient's immune system.

Dr. Gerald Epstein, a professor of psychiatry at New York's Mount Sinai Medical Center, has outlined dozens of imaging exercises in a book on healing visualizations. He describes one patient who credited her image of a broken bone knitting itself back together with healing her fractured wrist in three weeks instead of the anticipated three months. Epstein concedes that the rapid healing may have been a coincidence, but he believes he has witnessed similar results in too many other patients for coincidence to be the sole explanation.

People who are perfectly well can also benefit from imagery. For example, many athletes, dancers, and musicians resort to imagery to improve their performance; actors sometimes draw upon it to overcome stage fright or help remember their lines.

Music Therapy

In this treatment, music and rhythm are used to improve physical and psychological functioning and provide an alternative means of communication for persons who are unable to put their feelings or thoughts into words.

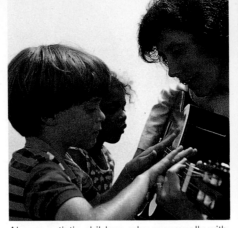
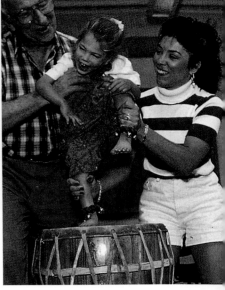

Above, autistic children, who are usually withdrawn, respond to a guitar. At right, a blind, multiply handicapped child learns alternate stepping with the help of rhythmic music.

Origins
Music therapy probably began when the earliest humans stomped or clapped to invoke healing spirits or to exorcise a sick person's demons. Greek myths contain metaphors for the healing power of music, and musical cures were part of many ancient cultures and religions.

More recently, a number of health professionals have adopted music therapy in their practices. One doctor noted for his work in this field is Oliver Sacks, a New York neurologist and the author of *Awakenings*, who recognized the healing power of music in 1969 when working with catatonic patients. His 1973 book, later made into a movie, described how music therapy helped many of these patients adjust to the world after years as catatonics. At the Rusk Institute for Rehabilitation Medicine in New York, music therapy is used to treat patients with physical and/or mental disabilities.

Practitioners
In Canada, accredited music therapists must have completed courses at Wilfrid Laurier University, home to the Canadian Music Therapy Association. Similar courses are also offered at Windsor University, Capilano College (Vancouver), and Université du Québec à Montréal.

When it is used
Music therapy encompasses three major subdivisions:

Medicine: In this practice, music is used to help manage organic disorders, such as pain, and for rehabilitation after a stroke or a serious accident. The aged and patients with Parkinson's disease improve coordination and learn to walk with a steadier gait by exercising to music. Singing or playing certain musical instruments may contribute to improved lung function. Singing is also used to overcome speech disorders.

Psychotherapy: Music, as a universal language, can help psychotherapists to communicate with patients who are unable to verbalize their problems. It is especially beneficial in treating autistic and emotionally disturbed children.

Special education: In this application, music helps improve the coordination of children with neurological disabilities, as well as those who are blind or deaf. When incorporated into group activities, it also contributes to socialization.

How it works
The healing effects of music on all aspects of mind/body function are universally accepted but not scientifically understood. Some researchers believe that music reaches a part of the brain that is not involved with verbal skills. For example, old songs often spark remarkable responses from Alzheimer's patients. Some researchers believe that music activates a flow of stored memory that is otherwise inaccessible.

Research suggests that musical experiences may also trigger the production of endorphins, brain chemicals that are natural painkillers. Studies by anesthesiologists indicate that playing music during surgery reduces the need for anesthesia. Dentists have also observed that their patients don't need as much painkiller when music is being played.

What to expect
Activities may proceed on a one-to-one basis or in a group, depending on the desired result. Participants join in actively or listen passively. For example, a young group may drum rhythmically or exercise to jazz, while geriatric patients may listen to music that was popular during their younger years.

A DRAMATIC ROUTE TO HEALING
To most of us, play acting is little more than a flight of fancy. But to the emotionally disturbed or developmentally handicapped, drama, used as therapy (an outgrowth of music therapy), is a valuable method in the healing process. The goal is to enable a person to experiment with thoughts and emotions in a nonthreatening setting. By assuming a dramatic role, many people can act out emotions they would be unable to express otherwise.

Drama therapy is especially effective in settings where individuals have difficulty relating to each other; for example, in schools for emotionally disturbed children. It is also used in prisons and in programs for those who have difficulty living in society.

In some instances, the patients create their own dramas, but more commonly, a drama therapist draws upon a familiar story, such as a fairy tale, that can be applied to the situation at hand. The therapist then observes how the various players interpret their roles, and in later sessions uses the drama as a basis for discussing their own problems.

In other situations, drama therapy may be used to build a sense of self-worth. For example, schoolchildren from minority groups may be encouraged to put on a play for their classmates that depicts some special event in their history or aspect of their cultural heritage. This exercise can be educational for the audience as well as therapeutic for the actors.

Precautions
▶ Check the qualifications of a music therapist before beginning a course of treatment. The Canadian Association for Music Therapy (Wilfrid Laurier University, Waterloo ON N2L 3C5) maintains a list of accredited music therapists.

Naturopathy and Natural Healing

Naturopathy is based on natural means of healing diseases. Its practitioners often employ the entire spectrum of alternative therapies. Instead of conventional drugs, for example, they may choose from among herbal medicines, homeopathic remedies, nutrition and diet therapy, acupuncture, hydrotherapy, and physical therapy.

Naturopaths describe themselves as holistic practitioners who rely heavily on patient counseling and education. They also include among their treatments some practices of conventional medicine. For instance, they may use diathermy (a form of electrotherapy) for backaches. Many practitioners are also trained in techniques of behavior modification, such as biofeedback and hypnosis; others offer massage and other therapies for stress management.

Origins

Naturopathy originated during the 19th century, when a medical regimen based on hydrotherapy, exercise, fresh air, sunlight, and herbal teas gained a large following in Germany. The system was brought to North America by a German healer, Benedict Lust, who founded the American School of Naturopathy in New York in 1902.

Lust called for the elimination of "evil" habits such as overeating, the use of alcoholic drinks, tea, coffee, and cocoa, and advocated corrective habits of breathing, exercise, and a wholesome mental outlook. He also recommended good nutrition, periodic fasting, and various forms of hydrotherapy. He took a militant stand against "the drugs, vaccines, and serums employed by superstitious moderns" in favor of "natural forces much more orthodox than the artificial resources of the druggist," which he described as harmful and irritating to the human body.

Naturopathy quickly developed a wide following in the United States and Canada. But eventually, the practice could not compete successfully with modern medical and surgical techniques, nor could it deal with widespread accusations of quackery. By the 1960s, naturopathy had all but vanished from the scene. Today, however, this therapy is beginning to make a comeback.

Practitioners

The designation N.D. stands for Doctor of Naturopathy and indicates that the practitioner has completed studies in one of three naturopathy schools located in Seattle, Washington; Portland, Oregon; or Toronto, Canada. The course of study covers nutrition and various alternative therapies, including herbal medicine, homeopathy, Chinese medicine, massage, and manipulation. Hydrotherapy and other aspects of physical medicine are also studied. In Canada, naturopathic practitioners are licensed in British Columbia, Saskatchewan, Manitoba, and Ontario.

Some aspects of naturopathy and natural healing are also performed by acupuncturists, herbalists, massage therapists, nutritionists, and chiropractors, as well as by self-proclaimed healers with no formal credentials.

When it is used

While some people prefer a naturopathic practitioner as their primary doctor, others may visit one for specific treatments, such as hydrotherapy for arthritis or herbal preparations as

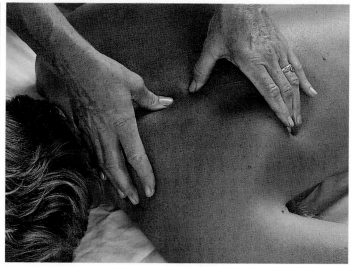

Naturopaths often incorporate massage and other hands-on techniques as part of their natural practices.

alternatives to pharmaceutical medications. Actually, some components of natural healing are used by most people as simple self-care: for example, a high-fiber diet to treat constipation, a warm bath to ease stress, exercise to alleviate depression, or self-massage for muscle aches.

How it works

The major premise of natural healing is that the human organism is capable of resisting disease and healing itself. Therefore the way to achieve wellness is to promote the body's self-healing capabilities. Naturopaths emphasize the responsibility of each individual in eating a sensible diet, exercising, and following a prudent, healthful lifestyle.

What to expect

The first visit is devoted to exploring the patient's medical history and lifestyle. After a diagnosis is made, the patient and practitioner evolve a holistic program. Here, for example, is a summary of the treatment for osteoarthritis as presented in the *Encyclopedia of Natural Medicine* by Michael Murray, N.D. and Joseph Pizzorno, N.D.:

Diet: Avoid all simple carbohydrates (sugars); stress starchy and high-fiber foods, and flavonoid-rich berries such as blueberries and raspberries; keep fats to a minimum; eliminate tomatoes, potatoes, eggplant, and peppers.

Supplements: Take niacinamide, methionine, pantothenic acid, zinc, and copper, and vitamins A, B_6, C, and E.

Botanical medicines: Use yucca leaves and extract and the powdered root of devil's claw.

Physical therapy and exercise: Include isometric exercises and swimming daily. Try short-wave diathermy and other physical therapy treatments that may be helpful.

Precautions
▶ When faced with a serious illness, such as diabetes or cancer, naturopathy should be approached as an adjunct to, not substitute for, conventional medicine.
▶ Be wary of any alternative practitioner who hesitates to refer any patient who has symptoms of serious illness, such as heart disease, diabetes, or cancer, to a medical doctor.

Nutrition Therapy

Nutrition therapy is based on the premise that diet in general or certain vitamins and minerals in particular can prevent or cure disease. Practices range from simply eating a balanced diet to maintain good health to taking megadoses of vitamins and/or minerals to ward off disease or treat mental illness.

A growing body of scientific evidence indicates that nutrition is even more important in preventive medicine than previously thought. But the majority of doctors and nutritionists still stress that for most people, a varied diet—low in fat and sugar, high in fiber and starches, and low enough in calories to maintain ideal weight—will suffice.

Origins

Physicians have been prescribing special diets since the time of the ancient Greeks, and they continue to do so for patients with nutrition-related diseases. The more recent practice of

megavitamin therapy (consuming at least 10 times the Recommended Nutrient Intakes, or RNI) originated with Dr. Linus Pauling, a Nobel laureate chemist who coined the term orthomolecular therapy (meaning therapy with the right molecules) in 1968, when he began to advocate very large doses of vitamin C to prevent or treat the common cold. During the 1970s, megavitamin therapy was promoted as an alternative treatment for mental illness. More recently, it has been advocated by food faddists and self-styled healers, as well as some conventional practitioners, as a cure for asthma, allergies, AIDS, and even cancer. Although good nutrition plays a role in treating these problems, there is no scientific proof that it can produce a cure.

Practitioners

In Canada, there are more than 5,000 registered dietitians who are members of the Canadian Dietetic Association. A dietitian must have a bachelor's degree specializing in food

ADULT RNI'S FOR MAJOR VITAMINS AND MINERALS

NUTRIENT	ADULT RANGE*	NEEDED FOR	SOURCES
FAT-SOLUBLE VITAMINS:			
Vitamin A	800-1000 RE**	Vision, reproduction, teeth, bones, hair, immune system	Dairy products, green or yellow vegetables, orange or yellow fruits, organ meats
Vitamin D	10 mcg	Bone growth and calcium absorption	Fish liver oil, liver, vitamin D fortified milk, egg yolks, sun
Vitamin E	8-10 IU‡	Making red blood cells and muscle tissue; preventing oxidation of fatty acids	Cooked greens, whole grains, seafood, poultry, eggs, seeds and nuts, wheat germ
Vitamin K	60-80 mcg	Blood clotting	Leafy green vegetables, potatoes, organ meats, grains
WATER-SOLUBLE VITAMINS:			
Vitamin C	60 mg	Immune system, healing, formation of bones, teeth, and blood vessels	Citrus fruits, tomatoes, green peppers, melons, broccoli, other fruits and vegetables
Thiamin	1.1-1.5 mg	Metabolism and nerve function	Seafood, pork, fortified cereals and breads
Riboflavin	1.3-1.7 mg	Vision and metabolism	Dairy products, organ meats, green leafy vegetables, red meats, dark poultry meat, fortified cereals
Niacin	15-19 mg	Proper nerve function; making digestive enzymes	Poultry, seafood, seeds, nuts, fortified cereals and breads
Vitamin B_6	1.6-2 mg	Formation of red blood cells; metabolism and nerve function	Fish, poultry, meats, spinach, bananas, cereals, sweet and white potatoes, prunes
Folate	180-200 mcg	Making DNA; formation of red blood cells	Liver, whole grains, fruits, legumes, dark green leafy vegetables
Vitamin B_{12}	2 mcg	Building genetic material; formation of red blood cells	Meats, eggs, seafood, milk, and milk products
MINERALS:			
Calcium	800-1200 mg	Bone and tooth formation; heart, muscle, and nerve function	Milk, milk products, green leafy vegetables, tofu, broccoli, canned salmon and sardines (with bones)
Iron	10-15 mg	Making myoglobin and hemoglobin	Liver, red meat, fish, dried apricots, legumes, soybean flour, raisins
Magnesium	280-350 mg.	Making digestive enzymes, DNA, and cells	Beans, oysters, scallops, fortified cereals, green vegetables
Phosphorus	800-1200 mg.	Tooth and bone growth; nerve and muscle function	Poultry, meat, dairy products, egg yolks, fish, legumes
Selenium	55-70 mcg.	Preventing oxidation of fatty acids in tandem with vitamin E	Seafood, egg yolks, chicken, mushrooms, garlic, onions
Zinc	12-15 mg.	Metabolism and the digestive system	Yogurt, beef, wheat germ, liver, fortified cereals

* Lower number is for women; higher for men, except for iron, which women require in the larger amounts.
**Retinol equivalent, the preferred unit of measure for vitamin A. One RE is equal to 3.5 IU from plant sources and 10 IU from animal sources. (Vitamin manufacturers measure vitamin A in IU.)
‡ Alpha tocopherol equivalents, the standard measuring unit of dietary vitamin E..

HIGH-DOSE ANTIOXIDANT VITAMIN THERAPY

NUTRIENT	MEGADOSE	UNPROVED HEALTH CLAIMS	POTENTIAL DANGERS
Vitamin A	15,000-25,000 RE per day	Reduces risk of breast, lung, colon, prostate, and cervical cancer; helps prevent heart disease and stroke; retards macular degeneration.	May cause liver damage, hair loss, blurred vision, headaches, fatigue, diarrhea, irregular periods, dry skin, benign skin yellowing, rashes, joint and bone pain. May lead to birth defects if taken during pregnancy.
Vitamin E	200-400 IU per day	Enhances fertility and improves sexual potency; retards aging process; helps prevent cancer and heart attacks; deters cataracts; relieves premenstrual syndrome and nocturnal leg cramps; protects against radiation damage from sun, air pollutants, and other environmental toxins.	Appears safe in recommended doses; may cause bleeding problems in rare cases of vitamin K deficiency or when taken with aspirin.
Vitamin C	250-1000 mg per day	Helps prevent cancer, heart attacks, and heart disease; bolsters immunity against colds and other infections; lowers blood cholesterol; protects against pollutants and environmental toxins; improves adaptation to stress; retards macular degeneration; deters cataracts; enhances fertility in men.	May cause excessive gas, diarrhea, urinary burning, mouth and intestinal irritation, damage to tooth enamel; can cause hemorrhages in patients with advanced cancer.

and nutrition, and also some practical experience, usually in a hospital or community setting. In addition, some doctors have passed qualifying examinations in this specialty.

The terms "Dietitian" or "Registered Dietitian" are protected by law to ensure only qualified people use these titles. The term "nutritionist" is not protected by law in all provinces. People with different levels of training and knowledge often call themselves nutritionists. In some cases, however, a qualified dietitian may use the term "nutritionist" in a job title. Depending on the province, "registered dietitian" is abbreviated as follows: RD, PDt, RDt, RDN, or, in Quebec, Dt.P. Your provincial dietetic association can direct you to qualified dietitians in your area.

Many chiropractors, naturopaths, herbalists, acupuncturists, health-club workers, and health-food salespeople also double as nutrition counselors.

When it is used

Dietitians are consulted to treat obesity, eating disorders, and diseases caused by deficiencies of certain vitamins and minerals. Although deficiency diseases are rare in the United States, they still occur, especially among the poor. The elderly and alcoholics are also vulnerable because they often consume very limited types and amounts of food.

Good nutrition has become an important component of treating diabetes, heart disease, and intestinal disorders. A dietitian may also be asked to recommend dietary changes for a hyperactive child or for a person with allergies, lactose intolerance, or metabolic disorders. Healthy people, such as athletes and pregnant women, also turn to nutrition therapists for dietary advice to meet their special needs.

High-dose vitamins are used in both conventional and alternative medicine, but for very different purposes. For example, very high doses of niacin (a B vitamin) are sometimes used in conventional medicine to lower blood cholesterol. High-dose vitamin E may be prescribed to treat fibrocystic breasts, and alcoholics may be given large amounts of thiamine. Alternative practitioners, on the other hand, recommend high doses of vitamins—the benefits of which are unproven—for a wider range of illnesses. Research indicates that beta carotene (a precursor of vitamin A) and vitamins A,C, and E (antioxidant

nutrients that offset harmful effects of oxygen metabolism) may help prevent cancer and heart disease and slow the aging process, but new data suggest that eating foods high in these nutrients is more effective than taking supplements.

How it works

Because vitamins and minerals are essential to normal metabolism and other body functions (see chart, opposite page), keeping a proper balance of them in the system is important to good health. However, a vitamin or mineral consumed in amounts greater than your body readily needs takes on the properties of a drug, and as with any drug, it carries a risk of side effects (see chart, above). For example, excesses of vitamins A and D, which are stored in the liver and fatty tissue, can lead to toxicity. High doses of minerals, especially iron, potassium, and lithium, can also be toxic.

What to expect

A dietitian will begin with a careful health assessment and a review of the patient's diet. If the person has a chronic health problem such as diabetes, the nutrition therapist should work with the primary care physician.

In cases that involve obesity or eating disorders, psychotherapy and behavior modification play an important role in long-term success. Some dietitians ask that clients keep a careful food diary; others inspect the client's kitchen shelves. Occasionally, nutrition therapists even show clients how to make wise choices at supermarkets and restaurants.

Precautions
► Never undertake to treat yourself or a family member with megavitamins. Vitamins in large amounts are powerful drugs with a high risk of unpleasant or lethal side effects.
► Keep vitamin and mineral pills out of children's reach. Iron overdose is a leading cause of poisoning death in children.
► Nutrition fraud is one of the most common forms of medical quackery. Be wary of any nutrition counselor who:
• Diagnoses deficiencies with hair or saliva tests (both worthless).
• Sells a private brand of nutritional supplements.
• Promises a nutritional cure for arthritis, asthma, or any other incurable chronic disease.

Pet Therapy

Pet therapy promotes human well-being through bonding with an animal, most often a cat, dog, or other household pet.

Origins

The domestication of animals and birds probably originated in prehistoric times. By the time the Egyptians exalted the cat to the status of a god about 3,000 B.C., household pets were common. In the late 1800s, the first seeing eye dogs for the blind were trained, utilizing the deep bond that develops between a sightless owner and an animal and inspiring the concept of pet therapy. In recent years, new therapeutic uses have been found for pets. This process began with an investigation of the contribution of pets to mental health. Since then, numerous medical studies have documented physical benefits as well.

Practitioners

Pet therapy may be initiated by a psychotherapist, physician, social worker, or family counselor. More often, it takes place informally, as when a parent gives a disabled child a pet to care for to help in building self-esteem, or an older person acquires a pet in order to cope with a loved one's death.

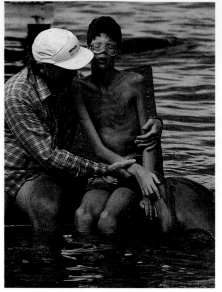

Dolphins are employed in a special education program for disabled children in Florida.

When it is used

Many situations are appropriate. Pet therapists have taken animals into nursing homes to be hugged and stroked by lonely residents who are usually unresponsive to those around them. Mentally disturbed, handicapped, and autistic children have received therapeutic benefits from touching and caring for a variety of animals, including horses and dolphins as well as household pets. Residential treatment programs for such children often involve some animal care. Also, a study at the Mayo Clinic found that cancer patients who were offered a companion cat while undergoing chemotherapy suffered fewer adverse side effects than patients who did not have an animal.

Prison rehabilitation programs sometimes include one-to-one involvement with an animal, during which participants may recall pleasures of childhood or enjoy for the first time a childhood pleasure they never had. Pediatricians have found that when there's a cat or dog in their office, children find a visit less threatening and are easier to examine. Dentists have noted that the presence of an aquarium in the waiting room eases the tension of anxious patients. Teachers often use animals to foster a sense of responsibility among young children.

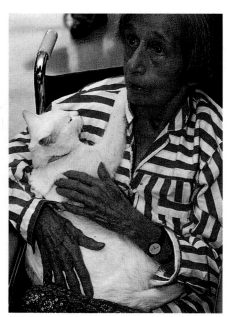

Holding or stroking a trusting animal helps a withdrawn person connect with a living creature, a critical step in establishing or restoring social interaction.

How it works

Every pet owner understands the rewards of having an animal that gives unconditional affection. But no one has yet explained why the companionship of a pet reduces heart rate and lowers blood pressure, or why elderly people who own pets make fewer visits to their doctor than those who don't. Numerous scientific studies have shown that pet owners also recover from surgery faster and survive a heart attack longer than those without pets. Some observers have noted that people who love their pets generally take better care of their own health because the animals depend upon them.

What to expect

Pet therapy takes many forms. Physically abused children, given the care of farm animals, may learn to express love for them which they themselves have not received. For a house-bound older person, the playful antics of a kitten or the purr of a contented cat might be a comforting distraction from pain. Dog owners can enjoy the health benefits of a daily walk and social interaction with other dog owners.

In a program at an upstate New York center for disturbed children, youngsters are allowed to care for injured wildlife and then release the animals to the wild after they have recovered. Dr. Samuel B. Ross, the initiator of this program, observed that: "It's an especially powerful experience for these kids who are, in a sense, wounded themselves. If you take care of a disabled animal and see that it can survive, then you get the feeling that you can survive yourself."

Precautions

▶ Don't give anyone an animal without first making sure that it will be welcome, and that the person will be able to care for it.

▶ If you're embarking on pet ownership for the first time, be sure to choose an animal that is compatible with your lifestyle. If you must work long hours, for example, you may have trouble caring for and training a dog.

▶ If you or a member of your household suffers from allergies, avoid getting an animal that has fur or feathers. In such cases, consider tropical fish or even an ant farm.

Spiritual Healing

Spiritual healing is the curing of disease through powers outside the limits of medical intervention. It is based on the concept that whatever one truly believes can be made to happen.

Origins

Virtually every ancient culture and religion believed that a specific person in the community was chosen by the spirit(s) to heal both physical and mental illness through supernatural powers. These healers were referred to as medicine men, priests, or shamans, and they were called upon to intercede with the spirits on behalf of their followers. For example, the Bible refers to miracles accomplished through faith and the transfer of positive thoughts from the healer to the sufferer. Whatever its origins, spiritual healing has always involved a belief in a universal healing force.

Practitioners

Spiritual healing is performed by people who claim to be endowed with the gift of thought or energy transference, which gives them a special link to a person in need of healing. One type of spiritual healing is practiced by Christian Scientists, who elect to treat themselves and their loved ones through prayer and faith in God, rather than depend on a physician. Alcoholics Anonymous and other 12-step support groups also rely heavily on spiritualism.

Therapeutic touch, which is practiced by countless conventional doctors and nurses as a routine part of patient care, is closely related to spiritual healing. Many observers believe that when a skilled, compassionate physician or nurse touches or clasps the hand of a trusting patient, an actual transference of healing energy takes place.

When it is used

Spiritual healers attempt to cure various acute and chronic diseases, including arthritis, cancer, diabetes, and even AIDS. Many people who go to spiritual healers for help have already exhausted the capabilities of more orthodox practitioners.

Precautions

▶ Because many people seek out a spiritual healer as an act of desperation, they are vulnerable to charlatans. While trust in the healer is a critical factor in the success of the encounter, financial commitments should be made with extreme caution.

How it works

No one can explain how spiritual healing works. Conventional physicians concede that there are hopelessly ill patients who miraculously recover, and in some of these cases, spiritualism is a factor. Spiritual healers contend that such cures are accomplished when patients become one with God (or with their own concept of a superior power).

Western researchers have studied psychic phenomena, including healing, in the United States and Europe, but they have yet to produce tangible results that are convincing to skeptics. Still, a growing number of conventional physicians, foremost among them cancer surgeon and author Dr. Bernie Siegel, are emphasizing the power of spirituality in the healing process. Most physicians report that patients who have a reservoir of spiritual faith tend to confront serious illness with unusual strength and calmness.

What to expect

Although some spiritual healers claim to have accomplished healing at a distance through the power of their thoughts, most practitioners work at the side of the patient. To prepare themselves for a healing session, they may spend time in prayer and meditation. Deep breathing, chanting, and other relaxation techniques contribute to the trance-like state that many healers enter for their work.

The healers remain passive until they feel they have been overtaken by healing power, which is then transferred to the ailing person. This transfer may be achieved solely through concentration, or it may involve a laying on of hands.

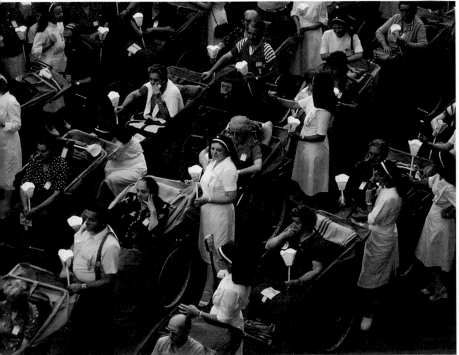

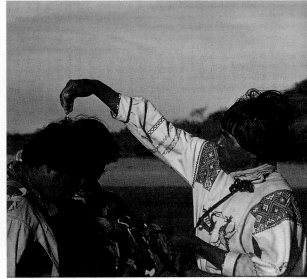

Native American shamans (below) continue to practice spiritual healing using the words and rituals of their predecessors. And each year, thousands of the faithful flock to Lourdes (left) seeking a miracle cure.

Yoga and Other Movement Therapies

Movement therapies employ structured exercise regimens and mental discipline to achieve both physical and emotional health. They range from the gentle approaches of yoga and t'ai chi to the more vigorous movements of aerobics and such martial arts as karate. They also include physical therapy.

Yoga emphasizes meditation, deep breathing, and pre-scribed body positions and movements. The martial arts incorporate meditation and structured movement as well, but the emphasis is more on self-control and self-defense. Despite the military aspects of these disciplines, they are rooted in nonviolence, with the goal of achieving mental and physical health. Aerobic conditioning has the additional aim of improving cardiovascular function, and physical therapy seeks to prevent or treat musculoskeletal problems.

Origins

Movement therapies trace their roots to ancient Eastern philosophy and practice. The term *yoga,* for example, comes from the Sanskrit word yuga meaning "to yoke" or "to join." Yoga practitioners, or yogis, believe that they can achieve cosmic union through movement and meditation.

Some people theorize that martial arts evolved from ancient dance rituals and meditative practices. Another theory, based on legend, holds that they began with Bodhidarma, the Buddhist monk who founded Zen Buddhism. According to this story, he taught young monks and was dismayed by their physical weakness, which he attributed to inactivity; so Bodhidarma developed ritualistic exercises to help increase their strength and stamina.

Practitioners

Yoga is taught in this country by physical therapists, physiatrists (specialists in physical rehabilitation), psychologists, and dance instructors, as well as by yogis and some of their advanced students. Many yogis are interested in transmitting all aspects of their way of life, including, often, pacifism and vegetarianism, through which they believe a spiritual unity with the cosmos can be achieved.

Martial arts are being taught mostly as a means of self-defense and building strength and coordination, but some instructors also emphasize meditation and spiritualism.

When it is used

Movement therapy is used to increase strength, counter stress, and control pain; devotees are all ages and come from every walk of life. Certain movements have been found effective in rehabilitation programs for victims of stroke or injury, and some yoga exercises have been adapted for the elderly and infirm so that they can be done in bed or in a wheelchair.

A number of psychotherapists have their patients learn yoga or t'ai chi to lessen anxiety and reduce panic attacks. Judo is sometimes recommended to help an overly shy child gain confidence and self-esteem.

Dancers and other performance artists use yoga and other movement therapies to overcome muscle tension and to limber up their bodies before rehearsals and performances. Dr. Dean Ornish, an American cardiologist, incorporates yoga in his innovative regimen for heart patients. At the Commonweal Cancer Help Program and research center in California, terminally ill cancer patients are taught yoga as a means of achieving serenity. The National Institute on Aging in the United States has been studying t'ai chi as an alternative therapy to help the elderly increase their fitness and mobility.

How it works

As currently practiced in North America, yoga, t'ai chi, and other movement therapies are viewed as a means of achieving mind/body harmony as well as physical strength. Performed regularly, they can help reverse the ill effects of a sedentary lifestyle, promote musculoskeletal strengthening of the body, and increase the suppleness of the spine. People who practice yoga or t'ai chi often describe a feeling of energy flowing through them. The breathing exercises of these therapies stimulate circulation while relaxing the body and mind. They also increase the capacity for focused concentration, and are often combined with meditation.

What to expect

Following is a more detailed description of what you can expect in a yoga or martial arts class. See boxes, opposite page, for aerobics and physical therapy.

Yoga. Instruction may take place one-on-one or in an organized class. Participants wear any attire that allows for freedom of movement. In general, shoes are not worn. During a typical beginning session, the instructor leads the class in a series of breathing exercises to warm up. A routine of stretches, bends, and other movements follows. The pace is usually relaxed and the movements flowing. Throughout the session, strong mental focus and deep abdominal breathing help participants maintain specific postures as long as possible.

T'ai chi. Instruction is usually given in a class, although some students opt for private sessions. Clothing that allows complete freedom of movement is appropriate, and comfortable, lightweight shoes may be worn.

Serious t'ai chi practitioners perform their routines daily. They execute the movements in a continuous, consistent, and somewhat slow rhythm. During the routine, all mental energy is focused on t'ai chi. The goals are to attain a mental state of complete calm and concentration, and to improve the technique continuously, thereby achieving both physical and emotional fitness.

Yoga combines meditation with breathing exercises and controlled movements to achieve well-being.

AEROBIC EXERCISE CONDITIONING

Aerobic exercise is any activity that requires extra oxygen and leads to improved cardiovascular function. Examples include brisk walking, jogging, stair climbing, swimming, and cycling. Such exercise forms the foundation for any well rounded fitness program.

Numerous studies have documented the value of aerobic conditioning: People who exercise vigorously on a regular basis live longer, have fewer heart attacks and other serious diseases, and enjoy a greater sense of well-being than their sedentary peers. Three basics are essential for a conditioning effect:

Frequency—three or four times a week.

Intensity—vigorous enough to increase your heartbeat to its target zone (see how to find it, right).

Duration—at least 15 to 20 minutes per session.

Some exercise physiologists add a fourth basic; *balance*. Excessive exercise can strain joints and supporting structures and increase the risk of sprains, stress fractures, and other injuries.

Designing an Exercise Conditioning Program

► Start with a physical checkup, especially if you are over the age of 40 or if you have any cardiovascular risk factors. These include a history of heart disease, diabetes, high blood cholesterol levels, high blood pressure, obesity, and a cigarette habit. A doctor may also recommend an exercise tolerance test to determine your safe level of physical activity.

► Next, pick an activity that you enjoy—if exercise is a drudgery, chances are you won't stick with it long enough to get in shape. Also consider what is appropriate for your age and general health. Almost everyone can undertake a walking program, whereas jogging, racketball, and high-impact aerobic dancing require not only stamina but also sturdy joints.

► Select the right equipment. Walking requires only well-fitted walking shoes and a safe, comfortable place to walk. If you would rather work out on a stationary cycle or other equipment, try it out before making an investment. If you are considering joining a health club, visit several and then sign up for a short trial period before committing yourself to a long-term membership. After a few sessions, you may decide this particular club is not to your liking.

► Start slowly and gradually build endurance. Many people do too much too soon, and end up with aching muscles and joints or more serious injuries. For example, if you are beginning a walking program, start by walking a mile at a comfortable pace. Over the next few weeks, gradually increase your speed and distance; for most people, two miles in 30 to 40 minutes is a reasonable goal.

► Include a few minutes of warm-up and cool-down stretching exercises before and after each session These help to prevent painful muscle tightness and injuries from overuse.

How to Find Your Target Heart Rate

Formula	Example for a 40-year-old
Subtract your age from 220	220–40 =180
Multiply the result by 75 percent	180 x .75=135

The result is the target number of heartbeats per minute. To find out if your heartbeat is in the target zone, exercise at peak intensity for 10 to 15 minutes; stop, find your pulse, and count the heartbeats for 10 seconds. Multiply by 6 to determine your heart rate.

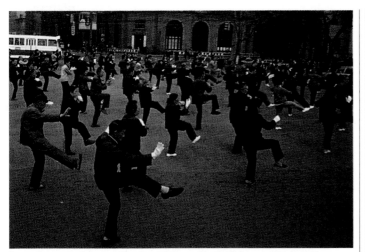

In parks and other public places throughout China, millions gather in the early morning to perform t'ai chi, an exercise ritual that the government has standardized with a routine of 24 movements.

Karate. This martial art is taught in a variety of settings, ranging from community centers to specialized schools. It is practiced barefoot, and traditional, loose-fitting white cotton jacket and trousers are usually worn. In a typical session, students meditate and stretch to warm up, then practice stances, kicks, punches, and blocks, controlling their movements with the help of deep, slow abdominal breathing. Finally, in unison, they perform formal exercises called katas.

Judo. Another hard martial art, judo is taught in most of the same settings as karate. Classes are also conducted in a similar manner, and the same type of clothing is worn. Judo students work on posture, balance, and judgment to perfect throws, falls, holds, and punches intended to disable attackers.

THE GROWING ROLE OF PHYSICAL THERAPY

Physical therapists are the health professionals most concerned with all aspects of movement, from restoring motion to joints that have been stiffened by arthritis to guiding novice athletes in techniques designed to prevent sports injuries.

Until fairly recently, most people consulted physical therapists only for rehabilitation following an injury or a debilitating illness. Now, however, healthy people who want to get the maximum benefit from exercise are consulting them for pointers on designing a program, avoiding injury, and managing minor problems such as muscle soreness. In addition, physical therapy is being employed increasingly in the management of both acute and chronic pain. In a sense, the field is bridging the gap between the medical disciplines of orthopedics, sports medicine, and physical medicine and the movement therapies such as yoga and the martial arts.

Physical therapy can be divided into three main categories:

► Preventive, in which a therapist helps develop low-risk fitness programs to prevent chronic diseases and such problems as lower back pain and tennis elbow.

► Treatment, in which a therapist designs individual programs for patients with specific injuries such as broken bones, or musculoskeletal problems such as chronic tendinitis.

► Rehabilitative, in which a therapist works over a long period with patients who have severe, debilitating conditions such as neuromuscular damage from a stroke or head injury. Rehabilitative personnel sometimes practice in tandem with occupational therapists, health professionals who help people with physical disabilities and movement disorders regain muscular control and find ways to perform the tasks of everyday living.

Physical therapists use several modes of treatment, including specialized exercises, electrical stimulation of nerves, hydrotherapy, heat and cold therapy, and massage. Sessions may take place in the patient's home, in a rehabilitation or physical therapy department of a hospital, or on the premises of an independent practice. Most health insurance policies cover a limited number of therapy sessions, if they've been prescribed by a physician.

Introduction

Taking charge of your own health care, deciding when to see a doctor, when an alternative practitioner might be more appropriate, and what you can handle yourself, is an intelligent, perhaps even necessary approach these days. Unfortunately, there are no easy guidelines—many physicians with years of training and experience often find such decisions difficult. Still, the more you know about how diseases can be treated, the more likely you are to make appropriate choices in managing your own and your family's medical care.

When to Call a Doctor

Tens of thousands of North Americans die needlessly each year because of denial and delay. Among them are heart attack victims who wait an average of six hours to call a doctor, and other people who ignore for months the common warning signs of a major disease such as cancer.

By contrast, those who run to a medical specialist for every ache, pain, and sniffle not only drive up medical costs, but also increase their risk of adverse reactions from overtreatment. The ideal is to find a middle ground based on common sense and knowledge.

Whom to See

As stressed in the previous section, everyone should have a primary-care physician to oversee and coordinate medical care. This might be a family practitioner, an internist, an osteopath, a pediatrician (for children), or a gynecologist (for women). The doctor may have his or her own practice or be part of a group practice or a clinic. The important thing is that your practitioner know your medical history and have a stake in maintaining your health.

When you are injured or acute illness strikes, always turn first to a conventionally trained medical doctor. These practitioners are the best qualified to treat trauma and other emergencies, infections, diabetes, heart disease, cancer, and other serious illnesses.

If you suffer from a chronic pain syndrome or some other condition for which conventional medicine can do little, you might be better off seeing an alternative practitioner. And in many cases, you may be the best person to manage your illness, often under the guidance of a medical professional.

In the box to the right and on the next two pages is a listing of medical signs and symptoms and their possible causes. The remainder of the section describes more than 450 diseases and conditions, both common and rare, and provides information on how they are treated, not only by mainstream physicians but also by alternative practitioners and with self-care. It also details how disorders are diagnosed and lists some important questions you should ask the health professional to whom you entrust your medical care. The goal is to help you make informed decisions about your well being.

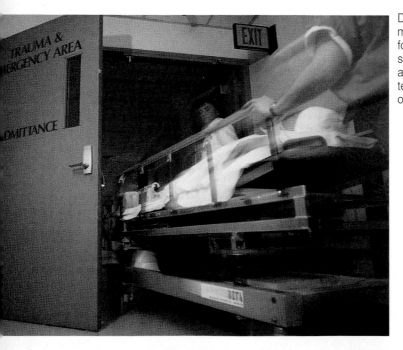

Delays in seeking medical attention for serious problems such as heart attacks are responsible for tens of thousands of deaths each year.

PROBLEMS THAT DEMAND PROMPT MEDICAL ATTENTION

Call your local emergency service or get to the nearest emergency room if any of the following develop:

Possible heart attack:
▶ Severe pain, lightheadedness, fainting, sweating, nausea, or shortness of breath
▶ Feeling of pain, pressure, fullness, or squeezing in the center chest that lasts more than two minutes
▶ Pain spreading from the center chest to the shoulders, neck, or arms

Possible stroke or mini-stroke:
▶ Sudden weakness or numbness on one side of the body, usually affecting the face, an arm, or leg
▶ Sudden loss of speech, or difficulty speaking or understanding speech
▶ Loss of vision or dimness, usually in one eye or half of both eyes
▶ Unexplained dizziness, unsteady gait, lack of coordination, or falling
▶ Sudden severe headache unlike any experienced in the past
▶ Abrupt loss of memory or altered mental abilities

Possible shock:
▶ Cold, clammy, and pale skin
▶ Weakness and lightheadedness
▶ Rapid, weak pulse
▶ Rapid, shallow, and irregular breathing
▶ Agitation and feeling of apprehension

Possible anaphylactic reaction:
▶ Severe swelling, especially around the eyes, mouth, and face
▶ Weak, rapid pulse
▶ Difficulty breathing
▶ Possible nausea, vomiting, and abdominal cramps
▶ Bluish tinge to skin and nails
▶ Confusion, dizziness, possible loss of consciousness

Possible internal bleeding:
▶ Coughing or vomiting up blood, which may look like coffee grounds
▶ Blood in the stool or urine
▶ Bleeding from a body opening, such as the ears, nose, or mouth
▶ Abdominal swelling and tenderness
▶ Excessive thirst

Fevers:
See a doctor as soon as possible if:
▶ Body temperature rises to 100.5° F (38° C) in a baby younger than 3 months
▶ Body temperature rises to 103° F (39.4° C) in a child or adult of any age
▶ Body temperature rises to 101° F (38.3° C) and stays there for three days
▶ Low-grade fever recurs or persists for two or more weeks
▶ Fever of any degree is accompanied by severe headache, stiff neck, swelling of the throat, or mental confusion

Signs & Symptoms

In medical terms, a sign is any visible indication of disease—bleeding, a rash, or swelling, for example. A symptom is something you can feel, such as pain, fever, or nausea, and it may or may not be accompanied by a physical change. Below are common signs and symptoms and their possible causes.

COMMON SIGNS AND SYMPTOMS

SIGN OR SYMPTOM	POSSIBLE CAUSES
Anxiety	Alcoholism, panic attack, premenstrual syndrome, stress, a thyroid disorder
Belching	Gallbladder disease, indigestion, a malabsorption syndrome
Bleeding and bruises	
Gums	Periodontal disease, leukemia, vitamin deficiency
Eye	Diabetes, high blood pressure
Nose	A clotting disorder, high blood pressure, injury, nasal polyps or tumors
Rectal	Anal fissure, colon cancer or polyps, diverticulitis or other intestinal disorder, hemorrhoids, ulcers
Skin	Allergic reaction, anemia, a blood or clotting disorder, Cushing's syndrome, drug reaction, hemophilia, injury, leukemia
Sputum	Bronchitis, lung cancer, pneumonia, pulmonary embolism, throat infection, tuberculosis
Urine	Bladder infection, urinary tract cancer, kidney stone, prostate disorder
Vagina	Abortion or miscarriage, cancer, a hormonal disorder, infection, menstrual abnormalities, injury, polyps
Vomit	Cirrhosis of the liver, esophageal tear, ulcers
Breathlessness	Anemia, anxiety, asthma, heart disease, hyperventilation, a lung disorder
Confusion	Addiction, alcoholism, Alzheimer's disease or other dementia, drug reaction, head injury, stroke
Constipation	Appendicitis, colon cancer or other bowel disorder, diabetes, diet, drug side effects, inactivity, pregnancy, a thyroid disorder
Coughing	Asthma, bronchitis, common cold, croup, cystic fibrosis, flu, pneumonia
Cyanosis (bluish skin)	A circulatory disorder, congenital heart defect, cystic fibrosis, heart failure, respiratory failure, Raynaud's disease
Delirium	Alcohol or drug abuse, brain tumor or abscess, encephalitis, head injury, heat stroke, meningitis, mountain sickness, poisoning, psychosis, Reye's syndrome
Diarrhea	AIDS, allergies, celiac disease, food poisoning, inflammatory bowel disease, irritable bowel syndrome or other colon disorder, infection, a malabsorption syndrome, traveler's diarrhea
Dizziness	Alcohol or drug abuse, anemia, a brain disorder, cardiac arrhythmia, drug reaction, ear infection, Ménière's disease, stroke or mini-stroke, tumor

SIGN OR SYMPTOM	POSSIBLE CAUSES
Fatigue	Anemia, cancer, chronic fatigue syndrome, depression, flu or other infectious disorder, heart disease, hepatitis, mononucleosis, premenstrual syndrome, respiratory disorders
Fever	Abscess, AIDS, appendicitis, cancer, infection (bacterial or viral), medication side effects, rheumatoid arthritis or other autoimmune diseases
Fainting	Anxiety, blood loss, cardiac arrhythmias, heart attack or other heart condition, hyperventilation, hypoglycemia, stroke
Gait changes	Arthritis, a back disorder, multiple sclerosis or other neuromuscular disorder, Parkinson's disease, stroke
Hallucinations	Alcoholism, drug reaction, fever, schizophrenia or other psychotic disorder
Hirsutism	Cancer, Cushing's syndrome, drug side effects, hormonal imbalances, polycystic ovaries or other ovarian disorder
Hoarseness	Anxiety, asthma, bronchitis, cancer, common cold, croup, polyps, smoking, thyroid deficiency
Impotence	Alcoholism, depression, diabetes, drug reaction, multiple sclerosis, hormonal abnormalities, a nerve disorder, surgery for prostate tumors or disease, a thyroid disorder
Insomnia	Alcohol and caffeine use, anxiety or depression, drug side effects, a thyroid disorder
Intestinal gas	Colic, colon cancer or other bowel disorder, diet, indigestion, a malabsorption syndrome
Itching	Allergies, chickenpox or other rash, dry skin, eczema, fungal or other infection, liver disease, stress, vaginitis
Jaundice	Anemia, blocked bile duct, cirrhosis, hepatitis or other liver disorder, gallbladder disease, a pancreatic disorder, infant prematurity
Loss of appetite	AIDS, anemia, cancer, depression, a digestive disorder, drug reaction, an eating disorder, infection, loss of taste
Mood changes	Alcohol or drug abuse, depression or other psychological disorder, drug reaction, a hormonal disorder, menopause, premenstrual syndrome, psychological stress
Nausea and vomiting	Alcohol abuse, appendicitis, brain injury, drug reaction, ear infection, gallbladder disease, food poisoning, gastritis, glaucoma, heart attack, hepatitis, indigestion, infection, intestinal obstruction, Ménière's disease, morning sickness, motion sickness, ulcers, vertigo

SIGN OR SYMPTOM	POSSIBLE CAUSES
Nightmares	Alcohol or drug abuse, anxiety, depression, fever, post traumatic stress syndrome
Numbness or tingling	Bell's palsy, carpal tunnel syndrome, a circulatory disorder, neuropathy, Raynaud's disease, shingles
Pain	
Abdomen	Appendicitis, a digestive disorder, gallstones, hepatitis, intestinal disorders, menstrual cramps, pelvic inflammatory disease, tubal pregnancy
Back	Arthritis, muscle spasms or strain, osteoporosis, ruptured disk
Chest	Angina, an esophageal disorder, heart attack, heartburn, pleurisy, pneumonia, pneumothorax
Ear	Infection, foreign body
Eye	Conjunctivitis, glaucoma, foreign body, iritis, sinus infection, injury, sty, tumors
Face	Bell's palsy, dental disease, headache, shingles, sinus infection, temporomandibular joint disorder
Foot	Arthritis, bunions, corns or calluses, gout, neuromas, warts
Generalized aches	Flu, lupus, mononucleosis, rheumatoid arthritis, shingles
Head	Brain tumor, migraine or other type of headache, muscle tension, sinusitis, stroke
Knee	Arthritis, chondromalacia patella, infection, Lyme disease, strain or other injury
Leg	A circulatory disorder, fracture, muscle injury, phlebitis, shin splints
Mouth	Canker sores, cold sores, dental cavities, gum disease, infection
Neck	Arthritis, meningitis, muscle injury, slipped disk, stress
Joint / muscle	Arthritis, lupus, strain or sprain, tendinitis
Throat	Cold, flu, laryngitis, strep infection, tonsillitis, quinsy
Painful intercourse	
In males	Penile warts, prostatic or urethral infection
In females	Menopausal dryness, vaginitis, premenstrual syndrome
Palpitations	Anemia, anxiety, caffeine, heart disease, hypoglycemia, menopause, medications, premenstrual syndrome, a thyroid disorder
Rashes	Allergies, drug reactions, eczema, an infectious disease, lupus, rosacea, toxic shock syndrome
Runny nose	Allergies, common cold, sinus infection
Seizures	Brain tumor, drug side effect, cerebral palsy, epilepsy, fever, head injury, hypoglycemia, toxemia of pregnancy, meningitis, poisoning
Speech problems	Alcohol abuse, Alzheimer's disease, Bell's palsy, multiple sclerosis, stroke, Parkinson's disease

SIGN OR SYMPTOM	POSSIBLE CAUSES
Swallowing problems	Anxiety, diphtheria, an esophageal disorder, pharyngitis, strep throat, throat cancer, tonsillitis, quinsy
Sweating	Anxiety, drug reaction, fever, heart attack, infection, menopause, stress, a thyroid disorder
Swelling and lumps	
Abdominal	Cancer, heart failure, hernias, internal bleeding, intestinal gas, kidney failure, liver disease, pregnancy, uterine tumor
Breast	Cancer, fibrocystic condition, mastitis
Generalized	Anaphylactic reaction, drug reaction, heart failure, kidney disease, phlebitis, a liver disorder, thyroid disease
Joints	Arthritis, sprains
Skin or body surface	Abscess, cysts or other benign growths, cancer, edema, enlarged or obstructed lymph glands, ganglion, hives, infection, moles, warts
Taste changes	Bell's palsy, cancer, drug reaction, gum or dental disease, liver disease, loss of smell, pregnancy, a salivary disorder
Thirst	Diabetes, fever, heat exhaustion
Tinnitus (ringing in the ears)	Brain injury or tumor, cold or flu, drug side effects, ear infection, exposure to loud noise, Ménière's disease, earwax buildup, otosclerosis, vertigo
Tremor	Alcoholism, anxiety, Parkinson's disease, a thyroid disorder
Urinary problems	
Discolored urine	Bladder or kidney infection, kidney stones, liver or gallbladder disease, urinary tract cancer
Incontinence	Aging, Alzheimer's disease, a bladder disorder, nerve deterioration, spinal injury, stroke
Urgency	Bladder infection, bladder tumor, diabetes, interstitial cystitis, drug reaction, pregnancy
Painful urination	Bladder infection, gonorrhea or other sexually transmitted disease, kidney infection, kidney or bladder stones, prostatitis, urethritis, vaginitis
Vaginal discharge	Cancer, cervicitis, gonorrhea, vaginitis, pregnancy, premenstrual syndrome
Vision problems	Cataracts, detached retina, glaucoma, iritis, macular degeneration, mini-stroke, retinopathy
Weakness	Anemia, cancer, Guillain-Barré syndrome, heart disease, infection, liver disease, multiple sclerosis, muscular dystrophy, myasthenia gravis, rheumatoid arthritis
Weight changes	
Unexplained gain	Heart failure, kidney disease, liver disease, medications, toxemia of pregnancy, underactive thyroid
Unexplained loss	AIDS, anemia, cancer, diabetes, an eating disorder, infection, an intestinal disorder, malabsorption syndrome, ulcers
Wheezing	Allergies, asthma, bronchitis, emphysema, heart failure, lung disorders